MRCS SYSTEM MODULES: MCQs & EMQs

Andrew Williams BSc MBBS FRCS
Surgical Registrar
Bromley Hospital, Bromley, Kent

Christopher L H Chan BSc MBBS FRCS
Specialist Registrar in General Surgery
St. Thomas' Hospital, London

Tom Hennigan MBBS FRCS
Colorectal and laparoscopic surgeon
Bromley Hospital, Bromley, Kent

Lindsey Barker BSc MB ChB FRCS
Specialist Registrar in General Surgery
Kent and Canterbury Hospitals NHS Trust,
Canterbury, Kent

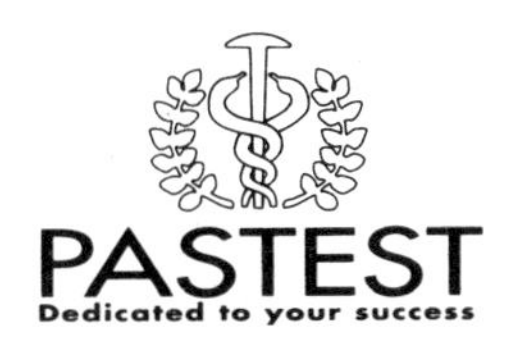

Egerton Court
Parkgate Estate
Knutsford
Cheshire WA16 8DX

Telephone: 01565 752000

First published 1998
Reprinted with revisions 1999

ISBN: 1 901198 103

A catalogue record for this book is available from the British Library.

Text prepared by Breeze Limited, Manchester.
Printed and bound by Biddles Ltd, Guildford and Kings Lynn.

CONTENTS

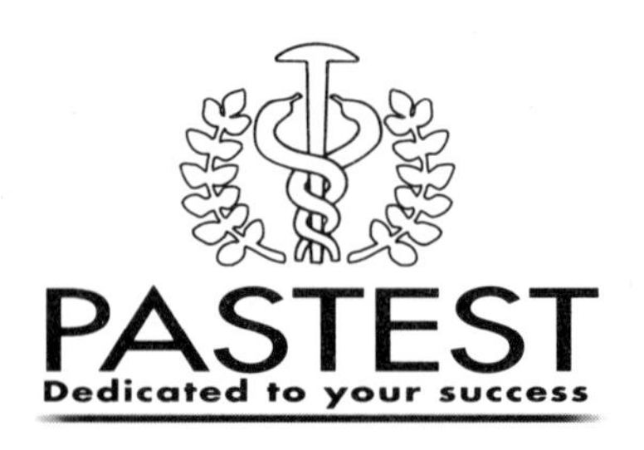
PASTEST
Dedicated to your success

PREFACE

The aim of the book is to help you pass the examination by helping you assess your knowledge and therefore alert you to the areas of your knowledge that require further study. It obviously cannot be a comprehensive textbook. However, the answers include a paragraph containing reasons why the answers are as they are and brief comments on the relevant surgical topic.

The authors have intentionally included areas of controversy. In these questions you may disagree with the answers but the aim is to stimulate further reading and discussion with your surgical colleagues. Not all of surgery is black and white.

Tom Hennigan

Acknowledgements

PasTest would like to thank Mr Steven J Walker, MD, MMedSci (Clin. Oncol.), FRCS (Gen. Surg.), Consultant Surgeon at the Blackpool Victoria Hospital, for his help with editing the manuscripts.

We would also like to thank Dr J P Garner for his assistance with reviewing the text.

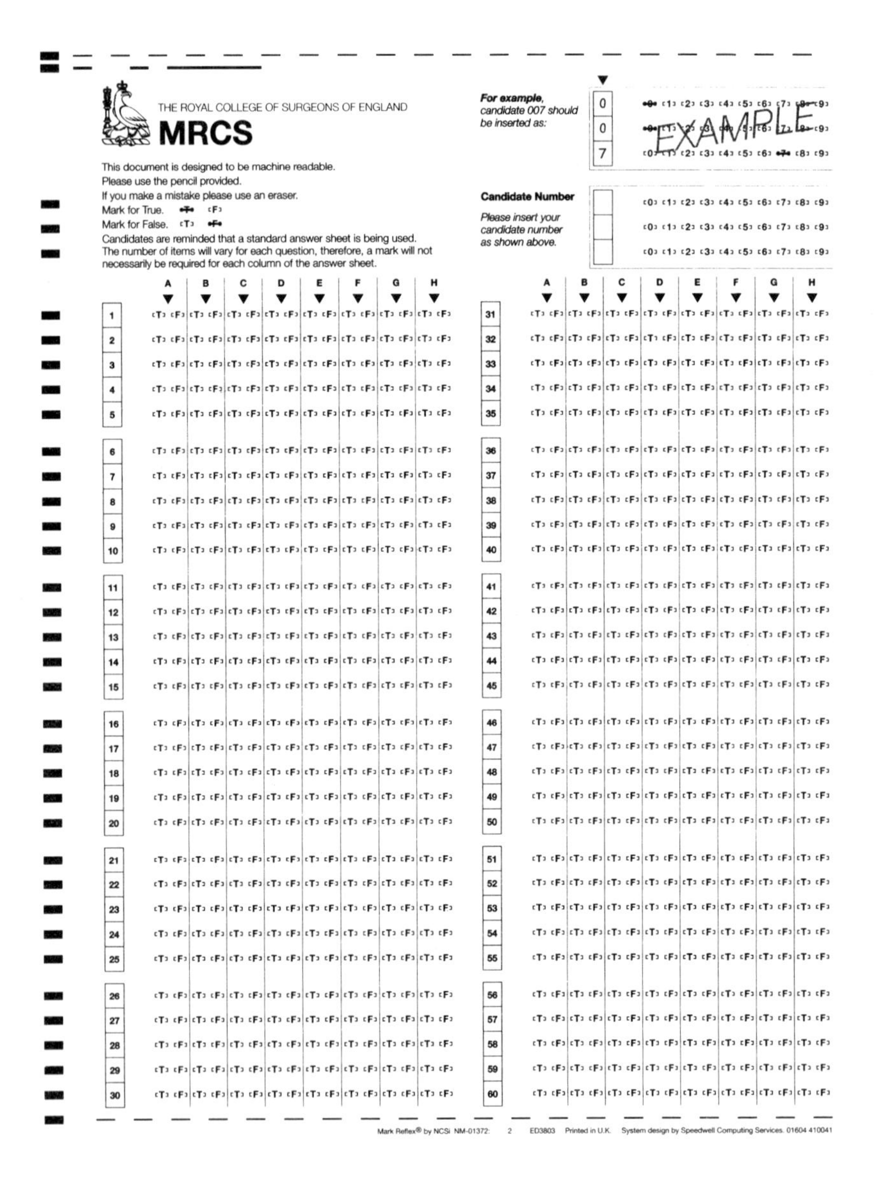

THE ROYAL COLLEGE OF SURGEONS OF ENGLAND

MRCS

This document is designed to be machine readable.
Please use the pencil provided.
If you make a mistake please use an eraser.
Mark for True. T F
Mark for False. T F
Candidates are reminded that a standard answer sheet is being used.
The number of items will vary for each question, therefore, a mark will not necessarily be required for each column of the answer sheet.

For example, candidate 007 should be inserted as:

0	0 1 2 3 4 5 6 7 8 9
0	0 1 2 3 4 5 6 7 8 9
7	0 1 2 3 4 5 6 7 8 9

EXAMPLE

Candidate Number

Please insert your candidate number as shown above.

	0 1 2 3 4 5 6 7 8 9
	0 1 2 3 4 5 6 7 8 9
	0 1 2 3 4 5 6 7 8 9

	A	B	C	D	E	F	G	H
1	T F	T F	T F	T F	T F	T F	T F	T F
2	T F	T F	T F	T F	T F	T F	T F	T F
3	T F	T F	T F	T F	T F	T F	T F	T F
4	T F	T F	T F	T F	T F	T F	T F	T F
5	T F	T F	T F	T F	T F	T F	T F	T F
6	T F	T F	T F	T F	T F	T F	T F	T F
7	T F	T F	T F	T F	T F	T F	T F	T F
8	T F	T F	T F	T F	T F	T F	T F	T F
9	T F	T F	T F	T F	T F	T F	T F	T F
10	T F	T F	T F	T F	T F	T F	T F	T F
11	T F	T F	T F	T F	T F	T F	T F	T F
12	T F	T F	T F	T F	T F	T F	T F	T F
13	T F	T F	T F	T F	T F	T F	T F	T F
14	T F	T F	T F	T F	T F	T F	T F	T F
15	T F	T F	T F	T F	T F	T F	T F	T F
16	T F	T F	T F	T F	T F	T F	T F	T F
17	T F	T F	T F	T F	T F	T F	T F	T F
18	T F	T F	T F	T F	T F	T F	T F	T F
19	T F	T F	T F	T F	T F	T F	T F	T F
20	T F	T F	T F	T F	T F	T F	T F	T F
21	T F	T F	T F	T F	T F	T F	T F	T F
22	T F	T F	T F	T F	T F	T F	T F	T F
23	T F	T F	T F	T F	T F	T F	T F	T F
24	T F	T F	T F	T F	T F	T F	T F	T F
25	T F	T F	T F	T F	T F	T F	T F	T F
26	T F	T F	T F	T F	T F	T F	T F	T F
27	T F	T F	T F	T F	T F	T F	T F	T F
28	T F	T F	T F	T F	T F	T F	T F	T F
29	T F	T F	T F	T F	T F	T F	T F	T F
30	T F	T F	T F	T F	T F	T F	T F	T F

	A	B	C	D	E	F	G	H
31	T F	T F	T F	T F	T F	T F	T F	T F
32	T F	T F	T F	T F	T F	T F	T F	T F
33	T F	T F	T F	T F	T F	T F	T F	T F
34	T F	T F	T F	T F	T F	T F	T F	T F
35	T F	T F	T F	T F	T F	T F	T F	T F
36	T F	T F	T F	T F	T F	T F	T F	T F
37	T F	T F	T F	T F	T F	T F	T F	T F
38	T F	T F	T F	T F	T F	T F	T F	T F
39	T F	T F	T F	T F	T F	T F	T F	T F
40	T F	T F	T F	T F	T F	T F	T F	T F
41	T F	T F	T F	T F	T F	T F	T F	T F
42	T F	T F	T F	T F	T F	T F	T F	T F
43	T F	T F	T F	T F	T F	T F	T F	T F
44	T F	T F	T F	T F	T F	T F	T F	T F
45	T F	T F	T F	T F	T F	T F	T F	T F
46	T F	T F	T F	T F	T F	T F	T F	T F
47	T F	T F	T F	T F	T F	T F	T F	T F
48	T F	T F	T F	T F	T F	T F	T F	T F
49	T F	T F	T F	T F	T F	T F	T F	T F
50	T F	T F	T F	T F	T F	T F	T F	T F
51	T F	T F	T F	T F	T F	T F	T F	T F
52	T F	T F	T F	T F	T F	T F	T F	T F
53	T F	T F	T F	T F	T F	T F	T F	T F
54	T F	T F	T F	T F	T F	T F	T F	T F
55	T F	T F	T F	T F	T F	T F	T F	T F
56	T F	T F	T F	T F	T F	T F	T F	T F
57	T F	T F	T F	T F	T F	T F	T F	T F
58	T F	T F	T F	T F	T F	T F	T F	T F
59	T F	T F	T F	T F	T F	T F	T F	T F
60	T F	T F	T F	T F	T F	T F	T F	T F

Mark Reflex® by NCSi NM-01372: 2 ED3803 Printed in U.K. System design by Speedwell Computing Services. 01604 410041

Sample answer sheet, reproduced by kind permission of the Royal College of Surgeons of England.

MCQ EXAMINATION TECHNIQUE

Before sitting an MCQ examination, you will need to know how many questions are likely to be on the paper and how long you will be given to complete it. Thus you will be able to assess the approximate amount of time that can be spent on each question. The time allotted for each of the written papers is **two hours**. Different questions are used each time, therefore subject composition is variable from exam to exam. There are approximately 45 MCQs questions and around 20 EMQs, depending upon the number of responses required.

Pacing yourself accurately during the examination to finish on time, or with time to spare, is essential. You must also decide on your own personal strategy for approaching the paper. You may decide to read quickly through the paper before picking up your pen, or to work slowly through the paper answering everything that you are certain of and leaving anything you wish to come back to.

There are two common mistakes which cause good candidates to fail the MRCS written examinations. These are neglecting to read the directions and questions carefully enough and failing to fill in the computer answer card properly. You must read the instructions to candidates at the beginning of each section of the paper to ensure that you complete the answer sheet correctly. You must also ensure that you read the question (both stem and items) carefully. Regard each item as being independent of every other item, each referring to a specific quantum of knowledge. The item (or the stem and the item taken together) make up a statement as "True" or "False". The number of stems will vary for each question. For this reason, a mark will not necessarily be required for each column of the answer sheet. For every correct answer you will gain a mark (+1). For the MRCS (London) examination, marks will not be deducted for a wrong answer. Equally, you will not gain a mark if you mark both true and false.

You must also decide on a strategy to follow with regard to marking your answers. The answer sheet is read by an automatic document reader, which transfers the information it reads to a computer. It is critical that the answer sheet is filled in clearly and accurately using the pencils provided. Failure to fill in your name and your examination correctly could result in the rejection of your paper.

Some candidates mark their answers directly onto the computer sheet as they go through the question, others prefer to make a note of their answers on the question paper, and reserve time at the end to transfer their answers onto the computer sheet. If you choose the first method, there is a chance that you may decide to change your answer after a second reading. If you do change your answer on the computer sheet, you must ensure that your original is thoroughly erased. If you choose the second method, make sure that you allow enough time to transfer your answers methodically onto the computer sheet, as rushing at this stage could introduce some costly mistakes. You will find it less confusing if you transfer your marks after you have completed each section of the examination.

You must ensure that you have left sufficient time to transfer your marks from the question paper to the answer sheet. You should also be aware that no additional time will be given at the end of the examination to allow you to transfer your marks.

If you find that you have time left at the end of the examination, there can be a temptation to re-read your answers time and time again, so that even those that seemed straightforward will start to look less convincing. In this situation, first thoughts are usually the best, don't alter your initial answers unless you are sure. Don't be afraid to leave the examination room once you are satisfied with your answers.

To guess or not to guess

Tests carried out at PasTest's MRCS intensive revision courses have proved that by far the majority of candidates can improve their marks by making sensible guesses.

The MRCS exams in England are not negatively marked[1]. For this reason you should answer every question as you have nothing to lose. If you do not know the answer to a question, you should make an educated guess - you may well get the answer right and gain a mark.

If you feel that you need to spend more time puzzling over a question, leave it and, if you have time, return to it. Make sure you have collected all the marks you can before you come back to any difficult questions.

Final advice

Multiple choice questions are not designed to trick you or confuse you, they are designed to test your knowledge of medicine. Accept each question at its face value, do not look for hidden meanings or catches.

The aim of this book is to enable you to evaluate your level of knowledge by working through the questions in each section. By marking clearly all of the answers that you got wrong or declined to answer, you can then refresh your memory with the explanations given here or read up on specific topics in depth using a textbook.

Working through the questions in this book will help you to identify your weak subject areas. Using books and lectures, you must work out your own personal profile of strengths and weaknesses and plan your revision accordingly. In the last few weeks before the exam it will be important for you to avoid minor unimportant areas and concentrate on the most important subject areas covered in the exam.

---

[1] The AFRCS examinations in Scotland are currently negatively marked.

ABBREVIATIONS

AAA Abdominal aortic aneurysms
ACE Angiotensin converting enzyme
ADH Anti-diuretic hormone
AFP Alpha-fetoprotein
AIDS Acquired immune deficiency syndrome
AKA Above knee amputation
AP Antero-posterior
APTT Activated partial thromboplastin time
ARDS Adult respiratory distress syndrome
ASA American Society of Anaesthesiologists
ATN Acute tubular necrosis
AV Atrio-ventricular
BKA Below knee amputation
BMI Body mass index
BP Blood pressure
CDH Congenital dislocation of hip
CEA Carcinoembryonic antigen
CMF Cyclophosphamide, methotrexate, 5-fluorouracil
CMV Cytomegalovirus
CNS Central nervous system
COPD Chronic obstructive pulmonary disease
CPAP Continuous positive airway pressure
CPR Cardio pulmonary resuscitation
CSF Cerebro spinal fluid
CT Computerised tomography
CVA Cerebro vascular accident
CVP Central venous pressure
CVS Cardiovascular system
DCIS Ductal carcinoma in situ
DIC Disseminated intravascular coagulopathy
DIP Distal interphalangeal
DSA Digital subtraction angiography
DU Duodenal ulcer
DVT Deep vein thrombosis
ECG Electrocardiograph
EDTA Ethylene-diamine-tetraacetic acid
EGF Epidural growth factor
EPL Extensor pollicis longus
ERCP Endoscopic retrograde cholangiopancreatography
ESR Erythrocyte sedimentation rate
ESWL Extracorporeal shock wave lithotripsy
ET Endotracheal
FAP Familial adenomatous polyposis
FDPs Fibrinogen degradation products
FEV_1 Forced expiratory volume in one second
FFP Fresh frozen plasma
FNAC Fine needle aspiration cytology
FRC Functional residual capacity
FVC Flow volume capacity
GA General anaesthesia
GCS Glasgow coma scale
GFR Glomerular filtration rate
GI Gastro-intestinal
GIT Gastro-intestinal tract
GMCSF Granulocyte macrophage colony stimulating factor
GORD Gastro-oesophageal reflux disease
GTN Glyceryl trinitrate
HCC Hydrocholecalciferol
HIDA Iminodiacetic acid
HLA Human leucocyte antigen
ICP Intra-cranial pressure
INR International normalised ratio
IPPV Intermittent positive pressure ventilation
IVC Inferior vena cava
IVU Intravenous urogram
JVP Jugular venous pressure
LDH Lactate dehydrogenase
LDL Low density lipoprotein
LH Luteinising hormone
LMWH Low molecular weight heparin
MCV Mean corpuscular volume
MEN Multiple endocrine neoplasia
MI Myocardial infarction
MIBG Meta-iodobenzyl guanidine
MNCG Multi-nodular colloid goitre
MRI Magnetic resonance imaging
MRSA Methicillin-resistant *Staphylococcus aureus*
MSU Midstream urine
NBSP National breast screening programme
NdYAG Neodymium yttrium aluminium garnet
NG Naso-gastric

NSAID	Non-steroidal anti-inflammatory drugs
PAN	Polyarteritis nodosa
PCA	Patient controlled analgesia
PDGF	Platelet-derived growth factor
PE	Pulmonary embolism
PEEP	Positive end expiratory pressure
PHPT	Primary hyperparathyroidism
PMC	Pseudomembranous colitis
PPIs	Proton pump inhibitors
PSA	Prostatic specific antigen
PSR	Peripheral sickle retinopathy
PTH	Parathyroid hormone
RA	Rheumatoid arthritis
RBC	Red blood cell
RTA	Road traffic accidents
RUQ	Right upper quadrant
SAH	Subarachnoid haemorrhage
SCC	Squamous cell carcinoma
SCD	Sickle cell disease
SLE	Systemic lupus erythematosus
TCC	Transitional cell carcinoma
TED	Thromboembolism deterrent
TENS	Transcutaneous electrical nerve stimulation
TIA	Transient ischaemic attack
TNF	Tumour necrosis factor
TPN	Total parenteral nutrition
TSH	Thyroid stimulating hormone
TURP	Transurethral resection of the prostate
UC	Ulcerative colitis
UICC	International union against cancer
UTIs	Urinary Tract Infections
VDRL	Venereal disease research laboratory
WBC	White blood cell
WCC	White cell count
WR	Wasserman reaction
ZE	Zollinger-Ellison

SYSTEM MODULE A: LOCOMOTOR

1.1 Late complications of fractures include

- ❑ A infection
- ❑ B Volkmann's ischaemic contracture
- ❑ C tendon rupture
- ❑ D myositis ossificans
- ❑ E algodystrophy

1.2 Fracture non-union

- ❑ A may occur if the fracture surfaces are interposed by muscle
- ❑ B characteristically produces painless movement at the fracture site
- ❑ C always requires treatment
- ❑ D may be treated by electrical stimulation
- ❑ E of the atrophic type may require bone grafting

1.3 The following are in keeping with a diagnosis of acute osteomyelitis:

- ❑ A bony pain
- ❑ B normal temperature
- ❑ C tenderness
- ❑ D normal X-rays
- ❑ E local inflammation

1.4 The following are features of rheumatoid arthritis:

- ❑ A Heberden's nodes
- ❑ B synovitis
- ❑ C normal ESR
- ❑ D early joint destruction
- ❑ E periarticular erosions

1.5 The following are extra-articular features of rheumatoid arthritis:

- ❑ A subcutaneous nodules
- ❑ B splenic atrophy
- ❑ C cutaneous anaesthesia
- ❑ D arterio-venous fistulae
- ❑ E renal failure

1.6 The following are complications of rheumatoid arthritis:

- ❑ A joint contractures
- ❑ B spinal cord compression
- ❑ C amyloidosis
- ❑ D malignant change
- ❑ E saber tibia

1.7 Delayed union of fractures

- ❑ A is rarely seen in the lower tibia
- ❑ B may be caused by intact fellow bone
- ❑ C produces a tender fracture site
- ❑ D produces a marked periosteal reaction
- ❑ E may be treated by functional bracing

1.8 Recurrent dislocation of patella

- ❑ A usually occurs towards the lateral side as the knee is flexed
- ❑ B is more common in varus deformity of knee
- ❑ C may give rise to osteoarthritis
- ❑ D has an equal sex incidence
- ❑ E is usually unilateral

1.9 Anterior knee pain may be due to

❑ A cruciate ligament injury
❑ B osteochondritis dissecans
❑ C torn meniscus
❑ D septic arthritis
❑ E traumatic synovitis
❑ F patellofemoral overload
❑ G collateral ligament fracture

1.10 The following clinical features may be indicative of the development of a melanoma in a pre-existing mole:

❑ A itching
❑ B decreased pigmentation
❑ C regularity
❑ D subcutaneous crepitus
❑ E satellite lesions

1.11 The following factors predict a good prognosis in malignant melanoma:

❑ A male sex
❑ B low Breslow thickness
❑ C the presence of ulceration
❑ D older age
❑ E a mucosal primary site

1.12 Acute septic arthritis of the knee

❑ A is most commonly caused by *Neisseria gonorrhoea*
❑ B is initially managed by aspiration and culture of the fluid from the knee
❑ C should be managed with non-weight bearing for six weeks
❑ D may cause locking
❑ E may lead to secondary osteoarthritis

1.13 Ankylosing spondylitis

- ❑ A is associated with HLA DR8
- ❑ B is more common in Africans
- ❑ C is associated with ulcerative colitis
- ❑ D may present as sciatica
- ❑ E often has a false positive rheumatoid factor

1.14 The following are X-ray features of osteoarthritis:

- ❑ A subchondral bone cysts
- ❑ B osteophyte formation
- ❑ C ankylosis
- ❑ D symmetrical joint space narrowing
- ❑ E periarticular osteoporosis

1.15 The following are true concerning bone formation

- ❑ A cancellous bone is dense and strong
- ❑ B woven bone is laid down in fibrous tissue
- ❑ C the shafts of the tubular bones are formed by lamellar bone
- ❑ D trabecular bone is less porous than cortical bone
- ❑ E cancellous bone is mainly found in the vertebrae and ends of long bones

1.16 Meniscal tears

- ❑ A more commonly affect the medial meniscus
- ❑ B occur when weight is taken on an extended knee
- ❑ C usually occur along the length of the meniscus
- ❑ D invariably heal spontaneously
- ❑ E produce localised tenderness over the joint line

1.17 Paget's disease of bone

- ❑ A characteristically only affects the cortex
- ❑ B can be treated with diphosphonates
- ❑ C causes an elevated alkaline phosphatase
- ❑ D is uncommon below 50 years
- ❑ E is most commonly found in the femur
- ❑ F predisposes to fractures
- ❑ G can be treated with calcium

1.18 A fall in serum calcium levels causes

- ❑ A reduced osteoclastic activity
- ❑ B increased vitamin D production
- ❑ C increased bone resorption
- ❑ D reduced PTH secretion
- ❑ E renal tubule impermeability to calcium

1.19 The following are true about calcium homeostasis:

- ❑ A calcitonin reduces renal excretion
- ❑ B calcitonin increases bone resorption
- ❑ C vitamin D is converted to 25 HCC in the kidney
- ❑ D vitamin D activation is increased by PTH
- ❑ E oestrogen increases calcium absorption

1.20 The following are causes of osteoporosis:

- ❑ A leukaemia
- ❑ B alcohol
- ❑ C tuberous sclerosis
- ❑ D hypothyroidism
- ❑ E hyperparathyroidism

1.21 The following are suitable investigations for metabolic bone disease:

❑ A plain X-rays
❑ B IVU
❑ C bone densiometry
❑ D iliac crest biopsy
❑ E MIBG scan

1.22 Congenital dislocation of the hip

❑ A has an equal sex incidence
❑ B is most commonly bilateral
❑ C is associated with acetabular dysplasia
❑ D should be investigated intially by ultrasound
❑ E may present in adulthood

1.23 Tuberculosis of the knee

❑ A may begin as a synovitis
❑ B rarely causes muscle wasting
❑ C causes subarticular bone erosion
❑ D produces a marked periosteal reaction
❑ E is usually diagnosed by acid fast bacilli in synovial fluid

1.24 Paget's disease of bone

❑ A is associated with sarcomatous change in 5%
❑ B is associated with cardiac complications
❑ C shows a decreased alkaline phosphatase
❑ D affects men more commonly than women
❑ E usually affects the upper limb girdle

1.25 The following are true about club-foot

- ❑ A the feet are held in equinus
- ❑ B the feet are held in valgus
- ❑ C the sexes are affected equally
- ❑ D it may be associated with neural tube defects
- ❑ E it invariably needs surgical correction

1.26 Acute osteomyelitis

- ❑ A is usually caused by *Streptococcus pyogenes*
- ❑ B may occur from a skin abrasion
- ❑ C usually begins in the metaphysis
- ❑ D is more common in the vertebrae in adults
- ❑ E has normal X-ray appearances during the first ten days

1.27 Post-operative osteomyelitis

- ❑ A often produces tenderness and pain on moving the limb
- ❑ B may be accurately diagnosed by MRI in the early stages
- ❑ C is more likely if there is implant loosening
- ❑ D is eliminated by prophylactic antibiotics
- ❑ E is usually due to a single bacterial pathogen

1.28 Carpal tunnel syndrome

- ❑ A occurs during pregnancy
- ❑ B is associated with hypothyroidism
- ❑ C characteristically produces pain during the day
- ❑ D produces a positive Froment's sign
- ❑ E may be diagnosed by nerve conduction tests

1.29 Hallux valgus

- ❑ A is associated with osteoarthritis
- ❑ B is usually bilateral
- ❑ C may be familial
- ❑ D responds well to splintage
- ❑ E may require joint fusion

1.30 Gout

- ❑ A most commonly affects the inter-phalangeal joint of the big toe
- ❑ B always has a raised serum urate level
- ❑ C may follow minor trauma
- ❑ D gives rhomboid crystals positive birefringence
- ❑ E may be secondary to myeloproliferative disorders

1.31 Complications of hip surgery

- ❑ A death
- ❑ B pulmonary embolus, no prophylaxis
- ❑ C urinary retention male
- ❑ D DVT, no prophylaxis
- ❑ E wound infection without prophylaxis

Match the post-operative risk with the complication for hip replacement.

1. 5–10%
2. < 1%
3. 1–5%
4. 30–70%
5. 10–20%

1.32 In the rheumatoid hand

- ❑ A ulnar deviation of the fingers is typical
- ❑ B a swan neck deformity refers to a flexion deformity of the proximal interphalangeal (PIP) joint
- ❑ C a boutonnière deformity refers to hyperextension of the PIP and flexion of the distal interphalangeal (DIP) joint
- ❑ D rupture of the extensor pollicis longus (EPL) is associated
- ❑ E Heberden's nodes are associated

1.33 Dupuytren's contracture

- ❑ A may be familial
- ❑ B has an association with carbamazepine therapy
- ❑ C often causes paraesthesia
- ❑ D should always be corrected
- ❑ E may require amputation

1.34 Humeral shaft fractures

- ❑ A usually require immobilisation in plaster
- ❑ B may cause weakness of the metacarpophalangeal extensors
- ❑ C are associated with delayed union
- ❑ D are uncommon in children < 3 years
- ❑ E take approximately four weeks to unite

1.35 Frozen shoulder

- ❑ A is usually due to impingement of infraspinatus
- ❑ B has painfree movement between 120° to 180° of abduction
- ❑ C has painfree movement between 60° to 100° of abduction
- ❑ D usually follows vigorous exercise
- ❑ E may be helped by a steroid injection below the clavicle

1.36 Perthes' disease

- ❑ A is common in Africans
- ❑ B is more common in girls than in boys
- ❑ C affects social class V more than I
- ❑ D has a peak presentation age at two years
- ❑ E shows a reduction mainly of abduction

1.37 A supracondylar fracture at the elbow

- ❑ A usually has the distal fragment displaced anteriorly causing brachial artery injury
- ❑ B is associated with compartment syndrome
- ❑ C usually leads to permanent damage to the median nerve
- ❑ D is associated with myositis ossificans
- ❑ E is commonly complicated by malunion

1.38 Combined fracture of the radius and ulna

- ❑ A in children is usually treated by open reduction and fixation
- ❑ B in adults usually requires open reduction and internal fixation
- ❑ C is commonly associated with posterior interosseus nerve damage
- ❑ D frequently causes ischaemia to the hand
- ❑ E may be complicated by cross union

1.39 Slipped femoral epiphysis

- ❑ A is complicated by avascular necrosis of the head
- ❑ B may lead to coxa valga
- ❑ C is more common in boys
- ❑ D commonly occurs at the age of 5 years
- ❑ E leads to a 'turned-in leg'

1.40 The following are risk factors for congenital dislocation of the hip (CDH):

- ❑ A female
- ❑ B polyhydramnios
- ❑ C sister had CDH
- ❑ D breech delivery
- ❑ E maternal alcoholism

1.41 A Colles' fracture of the wrist

- ❑ A is commonly associated with a fracture of the ulnar styloid process
- ❑ B unites in six weeks
- ❑ C is commonly associated with median nerve injury
- ❑ D may be associated with reflex sympathetic dystrophy
- ❑ E may cause shoulder stiffness
- ❑ F is associated with supination of the distal fragment

1.42 Internal fixation is

- ❑ A used in the treatment of pathological fractures
- ❑ B useful in the treatment of fractures in the multiple injured patient
- ❑ C occasionally complicated by chronic osteitis
- ❑ D used in the treatment of infected fractures
- ❑ E sometimes complicated by fracture non-union

1.43 Bone grafts

- ❑ A may take the form of chippings to fill a cavity
- ❑ B are commonly harvested from the ilium
- ❑ C are generally not suitable for splintage
- ❑ D do not produce an immunological response when harvested from another individual
- ❑ E donors are screened for HIV

1.44 Osteoid osteoma

- ❑ A occurs in the frontal bones of the skull
- ❑ B requires opiate analgesia
- ❑ C is best diagnosed on a bone scan
- ❑ D undergoes malignant change in 2%
- ❑ E is treated by radiotherapy

1.45 The following are true of bone tumours

- ❑ A brown tumours occur with thyrotoxicosis
- ❑ B aneurysmal bone cysts occur at the diaphysis
- ❑ C chondroblastoma occurs at the epiphysis
- ❑ D breast metastatic deposits are all sclerotic
- ❑ E prostatic secondary deposits are all porotic

SYSTEM MODULE B: VASCULAR

2.1 Calf claudication

- ❑ A is worse after a meal
- ❑ B is worse in hot weather
- ❑ C is worse walking uphill
- ❑ D may be accompanied by muscle spasm
- ❑ E may be present in the absence of significant atherosclerosis

2.2 Acute arterial occlusion is associated with

- ❑ A muscle wasting
- ❑ B cold limb
- ❑ C good collateral circulation
- ❑ D infarction of an end organ
- ❑ E bier spots

2.3 When acute ischaemia occurs in the lower limb the following are true

- ❑ A nerve function persists for up to three hours
- ❑ B striated muscle recovers well with minimal scarring
- ❑ C the hallucis longus muscle is the last to recover
- ❑ D in established cases compartment syndrome is rare
- ❑ E reperfusion of an ischaemic limb can cause cardiac arrest

2.4 Venous ulceration

- ❑ A may be associated with Klippel-Trenauney syndrome
- ❑ B should be managed by stripping the superficial varicosities in all cases
- ❑ C is more common in men
- ❑ D should be investigated by examination of the deep system in all cases
- ❑ E should not be biopsied as the cause is usually obvious

2.5 Ischaemic rest pain

- ❑ A is improved by dependent position
- ❑ B is most common in the calf
- ❑ C is a sign of minimal ischaemia
- ❑ D is worse in the afternoon
- ❑ E results in the area affected feeling cold

2.6 The following may suggest a diagnosis of mesenteric ischaemia:

- ❑ A abdominal pain ten minutes before food
- ❑ B profound weight loss similar to malignancy
- ❑ C bloody diarrhoea
- ❑ D calf claudication
- ❑ E vomiting after meals

2.7 The following are true concerning the spleen:

- ❑ A splenectomy may be indicated for leg ulcers
- ❑ B idiopathic thrombocytopenic purpura (ITP) is associated with the production of anti-platelet IgA by the spleen
- ❑ C hepatic failure is almost never associated with splenomegaly
- ❑ D sickle cell disease causes hypersplenism
- ❑ E may be enlarged in lymphoma

2.8 In primary lymphoedema of the legs

- ❑ A lymphatics in the epidermis are atrophied
- ❑ B malignant infiltration of inguinal lymph nodes is the most common cause
- ❑ C skin ulcers are uncommon
- ❑ D treatment with diuretics is of little use
- ❑ E lymph vesicles and fistulas usually require operative treatment

2.9 The following blood tests are suitable investigations for vascular disease:

- ❑ A packed red cell volume
- ❑ B erythrocyte sedimentation rate
- ❑ C VDRL
- ❑ D creatinine kinase
- ❑ E magnesium

2.10 The following are useful in the investigation of arterial disease:

- ❑ A plethysmography
- ❑ B greyscale ultrasound
- ❑ C thallium scanning
- ❑ D carbon monoxide delivery test
- ❑ E CT scanning

2.11 Carotid artery stenosis

- ❑ A of greater than 50% produces a 10% risk per year of stroke
- ❑ B is closely associated with coronary atherosclerosis
- ❑ C may be reliably diagnosed by auscultation alone
- ❑ D of greater than 90% is most easily diagnosed by duplex ultrasound
- ❑ E of 30–69% and symptomatic should undergo endarterectomy

2.12 The following are recognised surgical treatments for lymphoedema:

- ❑ A Homan's operation
- ❑ B lymphovenous microanastomosis
- ❑ C long saphenous vein transplantation
- ❑ D Trendelenberg's operation
- ❑ E mesenteric bridge operation

2.13 The following are compatible with rest pain but no gangrene in a foot:

- ❑ A Doppler index of 0.6
- ❑ B absent pulses below the groin on affected side
- ❑ C ischaemic ulceration
- ❑ D dorsalis pedis pressure of 40 mm Hg on Doppler assessment
- ❑ E biphasic pulse waveform at the posterior tibial pulse

2.14 Translumbar aortography

- ❑ A has up to a 1% mortality
- ❑ B may cause aortic rupture
- ❑ C is the most commonly used method to visualise the aorta
- ❑ D is commonly associated with anaphylaxis
- ❑ E utilises the Seldinger technique

2.15 Arteriovenous fistulae

- ❑ A may give a positive Branham's test
- ❑ B may ulcerate causing haemorrhage
- ❑ C usually improve in pregnancy
- ❑ D may cause multiple embolic events
- ❑ E are a feature of Klippel-Trenauney syndrome

2.16 Complications following carotid endarterectomy are more commonly seen in patients who

- ❑ A are male
- ❑ B are > 75 years
- ❑ C have ipsilateral external carotid stenosis
- ❑ D have a history of ischaemic stroke
- ❑ E have systolic hypertension

2.17 Indications for carotid endarterectomy include

❑ A symptomatic severe (> 70%) carotid artery stenosis
❑ B symptomatic moderate (30–69%) carotid artery stenosis
❑ C symptomatic mild (< 30%) carotid artery stenosis
❑ D large completed ischaemic stroke within preceding year
❑ E TIA sustained two years ago attributed to carotid artery stenosis

2.18 Routine clinical investigations in a patient with peripheral vascular disease are

❑ A serum cholesterol
❑ B serum autoantibodies
❑ C ESR
❑ D echocardiogram
❑ E plethysmography
❑ F ankle brachial pressure index

2.19 Strawberry patch

❑ A is a complex area of telangectasia
❑ B cases are 90% resolved by the age of three years
❑ C may calcify
❑ D may cause thrombocytopenia
❑ E responds well to a single treatment with cryotherapy

2.20 With regard to cervical rib

❑ A it most commonly causes arterial symptoms
❑ B a bruit may be heard in the supraclavicular fossa
❑ C paraesthesia is most common in the C6 nerve root
❑ D 70% are bilateral
❑ E it may cause digital gangrene

2.21 Traumatic bleeding

- ❑ A if large is best investigated by angiography
- ❑ B should be controlled by direct pressure
- ❑ C ligation in the field can be useful
- ❑ D may lead to distal thrombosis
- ❑ E should always be repaired with a vein patch

2.22 Arteriovenous fistulae

- ❑ A may cause limb lengthening
- ❑ B may cause valvular lesions
- ❑ C cause a bradycardia
- ❑ D may cause lipodermatosclerosis
- ❑ E may be iatrogenic

2.23 With regard to carotid endarterectomy

- ❑ A the untreated stroke rate of TIAs is 15%
- ❑ B surgery should be associated with a stroke rate of < 2%
- ❑ C the mortality from endarterectomy is 1–2%
- ❑ D a completed stroke is a contraindication for endarterectomy
- ❑ E surgery has been proven to be of benefit for stenoses > 50%

2.24 The following are used to monitor patients during a carotid endarterectomy:

- ❑ A proximal stump pressure
- ❑ B direct questioning of the awake patient
- ❑ C continuous MRI monitoring
- ❑ D transcranial Doppler
- ❑ E shunting during operation

2.25 In acute lower limb ischaemia

- ❑ A pain may be slight in the diabetic patient
- ❑ B sensorimotor impairment is the most important prognostic sign
- ❑ C sensorimotor impairment when present is irreversible
- ❑ D mottling with absence of blanching on pressure signifies microcirculation thrombosis
- ❑ E fasciotomy should not be used when revascularisation is planned

2.26 The following are associated with the formation of atheroma:

- ❑ A reduced PDGF levels
- ❑ B increased HDL levels
- ❑ C increased LDL levels
- ❑ D smooth muscle proliferation
- ❑ E oestrogen

2.27 Graft patency rates

- ❑ A reversed vein fem-pop graft
- ❑ B fem-pop dacron graft patency
- ❑ C aorto-fem patency
- ❑ D axillo-femoral patency
- ❑ E fem-fem cross-over patency

Match the following graft patency rates at five years.

1. 70%
2. 80%
3. 60%
4. 45%
5. 90%

2.28 Concerning amputations

- ❑ A toe amputations should be closed with 4/0 prolene in diabetes to avoid secondary infection
- ❑ B Chopart amputation is good for necrosis involving the heel
- ❑ C above knee amputations (AKA) should be 30 cm below the greater trochanter
- ❑ D Burgess below knee amputation (BKA) uses a skew flap system
- ❑ E rehabilitation is best after a below knee amputation

2.29 The common iliac artery

- ❑ A divides into the external and internal iliac arteries at the level of body of L5
- ❑ B lies anterior to the common iliac vein throughout its course
- ❑ C is posterior to the sympathetic trunk
- ❑ D is anterior to the ureter at its bifurcation
- ❑ E on the left is anterior to the preaortic autonomic plexus

2.30 The external iliac artery

- ❑ A becomes the common femoral artery after exiting the femoral canal
- ❑ B is anterior and then lateral to the external iliac vein before entering the thigh
- ❑ C is crossed by the ureter
- ❑ D gives off the inferior epigastric artery
- ❑ E enters the thigh midway between the anterior superior iliac spine and the symphysis pubis

2.31 The femoral sheath

- ❑ A contains the femoral artery in its medial compartment
- ❑ B has its lateral wall pierced by the genitofemoral nerve
- ❑ C has the greater saphenous vein piercing its medial wall
- ❑ D is a continuation of the fascia transversalis anteriorly
- ❑ E contains the femoral nerve

2.32 The following are true concerning aneurysms:

- ❑ A the elective mortality for abdominal aortic repair should be < 15%
- ❑ B surgery is of proven benefit for aortic aneurysms of 4 cm
- ❑ C the commonest peripheral artery aneurysm is femoral
- ❑ D splenic artery aneurysms are more common in women
- ❑ E in abdominal aneurysms 1–2% are supra-renal

2.33 Raynaud's phenomenon may be associated with the following:

- ❑ A dysphagia
- ❑ B occupation
- ❑ C warm agglutinins
- ❑ D cutaneous discolouration
- ❑ E Buerger's disease

2.34 The femoral artery

- ❑ A passes into the adductor canal deep to sartorius
- ❑ B lies on the muscles of the iliopsoas, adductor longus and adductor brevis muscles
- ❑ C gives off the profunda femoris artery from its medial side
- ❑ D contributes to the blood supply of the buttock
- ❑ E becomes the popliteal artery after passing through an opening in the adductor magnus
- ❑ F passes medial to the femoral vein

2.35 Principles of management of the diabetic foot include

- ❑ A tight control of the diabetes
- ❑ B topical antibiotics
- ❑ C removal of all necrotic tissue
- ❑ D drainage of collections of pus
- ❑ E protection of the other foot

2.36 The following are true of acute arterial embolism:

- ❑ A all patients must have a cardiac echo
- ❑ B thrombolysis has been shown to be superior to embolectomy
- ❑ C saddle thrombus usually needs an aortotomy to remove it
- ❑ D arteriotomy site should be closed with 4/0 polydioxanone suture
- ❑ E on table angiography is useful during embolectomy

2.37 Glomus tumours

- ❑ A are usually painless
- ❑ B are more common in men
- ❑ C are blue in colour
- ❑ D may cause phalyngeal changes on X-ray
- ❑ E are treated with radiotherapy

2.38 Match the following

- ❑ A Kaposi's sarcoma
- ❑ B angiosarcoma
- ❑ C chemodectoma
- ❑ D glomus jugulare tumour
- ❑ E leiomyomas

Match the most appropriate feature above with the list below.

1. carotid artery
2. more common in veins than arteries
3. rapid growing, bulky
4. blue/red macule with HIV
5. buzzing sensation in head

2.39 Varicose veins are associated with the following:

- ❑ A deep vein thrombosis
- ❑ B ulceration
- ❑ C ankle swelling
- ❑ D paraesthesia in the gaiter area
- ❑ E bleeding

2.40 Arterial stenosis

- ❑ A of 50% produces a 25% decline in flow rate
- ❑ B produces turbulence by reducing the velocity of blood flow through the constriction
- ❑ C in the lower limb is most common in the superficial femoral artery

2.41 The popliteal fossa

- ❑ A is covered by deep fascia beneath which runs the short saphenous vein
- ❑ B is formed medially by the biceps femoris muscle
- ❑ C contains the common peroneal nerve passing down lateral to the semimembranosus muscle
- ❑ D contains sensory nerves to the lateral side of the foot and ankle
- ❑ E has the popliteal artery deep to the popliteal vein

2.42 Major lower limb amputation

- ❑ A is associated with high incidence of DVT
- ❑ B should be covered by prophylactic antibiotics
- ❑ C is best performed with a tourniquet
- ❑ D in conjunction with pre-op epidural reduces the incidence of phantom limb pain
- ❑ E is always performed with equal skin flaps

2.43 Abdominal aortic aneurysm

- ❑ A are infra-renal in 80% cases
- ❑ B are associated with direct inguinal hernia
- ❑ C are associated with hypertension
- ❑ D are best assessed by arteriography
- ❑ E measuring greater than 5 cm should be repaired electively

2.44 Popliteal artery aneurysm

- ❑ A is a rare site for aneurysm formation
- ❑ B usually presents as a pulsatile mass
- ❑ C is associated with atherosclerosis
- ❑ D may be treated by resection and bypass grafting
- ❑ E may cause ankle oedema

2.45 The following are true of varicose veins:

- ❑ A some are truly congenital
- ❑ B simple veins post DVT need no investigation
- ❑ C may be only due to perforator disease
- ❑ D venous duplex Doppler is helpful in assessment
- ❑ E venograms are no longer indicated in the assessment

2.46 Venous ulcers

- ❑ A have a raised edge
- ❑ B may heal with conservative treatment alone
- ❑ C rarely undergo malignant change
- ❑ D have a positive WR test
- ❑ E are associated with Klippel-Trenauney syndrome

2.47 Deep vein thrombosis

- ❑ A is more common in smokers
- ❑ B is more common in patients with malignancy
- ❑ C may be diagnosed on ascending venography
- ❑ D may be diagnosed on B-mode ultrasound
- ❑ E may be diagnosed on thermography

2.48 Routine investigation of recurrent TIA should include

- ❑ A ESR
- ❑ B duplex Doppler of carotid arteries
- ❑ C intra-arterial subtraction arteriogram if heterogeneous plaque is noted
- ❑ D selective catheterisation of common carotid artery
- ❑ E CT brain

2.49 The external carotid artery

- ❑ A gives off the superior thyroid artery near its origin
- ❑ B lies deep to the hypoglossal nerve
- ❑ C divides into the superficial temporal and maxillary arteries distal to the parotid gland
- ❑ D has occipital artery at the level of the lower and upper borders of stylohyoid muscle
- ❑ E has posterior auricular artery at the level of the lower and upper borders of stylohyoid muscle
- ❑ F supplies the meninges

2.50 Femoral artery aneurysm

- ❑ A usually presents with pain
- ❑ B should be repaired if > 4 cm diameter
- ❑ C repair may be complicated by lymphatic fistula
- ❑ D is associated with aortic aneurysm

2.51 The following factors increase the risk of DVT:

- ❑ A elevated protein S
- ❑ B varicose veins
- ❑ C aspirin
- ❑ D oral contraceptive pill
- ❑ E sickle cell anaemia

SYSTEM MODULE C: HEAD, NECK, ENDOCRINE AND PAEDIATRIC

3.1 Tumours of the thyroid region may be monitored using the following:

- ❑ A calcitonin
- ❑ B serum calcium
- ❑ C ultrasound
- ❑ D sestaMIBI scan
- ❑ E parathyroid hormone

3.2 Cleft lip

- ❑ A affects boys more than girls
- ❑ B affects 1 in 750 live births
- ❑ C has an incidence which is on the decline
- ❑ D occurs with palatal defects in about half of cases
- ❑ E risk in subsequent children after a previous child is affected is 25%

3.3 Cleft palate

- ❑ A is associated with cleft lip
- ❑ B may causes hearing loss
- ❑ C repair results in speech recovery in only half of cases
- ❑ D cases may have teeth absent at the site of the cleft
- ❑ E should be repaired around three years of age

3.4 In the assessment of thyroid enlargement

- ❑ A fine needle aspiration cytology (FNAC) can accurately diagnose a colloid nodule
- ❑ B FNAC can accurately distinguish between a benign and a malignant follicular neoplasm
- ❑ C ^{123}I isotope scan is very helpful in the diagnosis of malignancy
- ❑ D ultrasonography can discriminate benign from malignant disease
- ❑ E MIBG (meta-iodobenzyl guanidine) may be useful in evaluating medullary thyroid carcinoma

3.5 On inspecting the dissected neck of a patient with primary hyperparathyroidism

- ❑ A a normal parathyroid gland would appear pinkish-red
- ❑ B the superior parathyroid glands lie behind the middle third of the thyroid lobes
- ❑ C the inferior parathyroid glands lie superior to the inferior thyroid artery
- ❑ D all four parathyroid glands are usually enlarged
- ❑ E flecks of ectopic calcification are frequently seen in the fatty tissues

3.6 Tumours of the hypothalamus

- ❑ A affect the appetite
- ❑ B alter mood
- ❑ C obstruct CSF drainage
- ❑ D interfere with temperature control
- ❑ E result in chiasmal compression

3.7 The presenting symptoms of cranial tumours include

- ❑ A nocturnal headache exacerbated by coughing
- ❑ B alteration of mood
- ❑ C diplopia on lateral gaze
- ❑ D apnoeic attack
- ❑ E vomiting

3.8 Carcinoma of the parotid gland is

- ❑ A the most common malignant tumour of the salivary glands
- ❑ B a recognised complication of pleomorphic adenoma
- ❑ C a recognised cause of facial nerve palsy
- ❑ D a radio resistant tumour
- ❑ E associated with a 10-year survival of 50% for high grade tumours

3.9 Match the following:

- ❑ A *Herpes simplex*
- ❑ B candidiasis
- ❑ C beta haemolytic streptococcus
- ❑ D fusospirochaetal infection
- ❑ E *Treponema pallidum*

Match the organisms above with the condition below.

1. Vincent's angina
2. gumma
3. cold sore
4. Ludwig's angina
5. thrush

3.10 Squamous cell carcinoma of the mouth is associated with

- ❑ A cigarette smoking
- ❑ B syphilis
- ❑ C alcohol
- ❑ D male preponderance
- ❑ E increased incidence in India

3.11 Papillary carcinoma of the thyroid

- ❑ A has a strong association with previous radiation exposure
- ❑ B secretes calcitonin
- ❑ C is found in iodine poor areas
- ❑ D is frequently multifocal
- ❑ E usually presents with distant metastases
- ❑ F is treated with thyroxine following total thyroidectomy to suppress TSH levels
- ❑ G is a disease of the elderly

3.12 Cancer of the lip

- ❑ A has a higher incidence among blacks
- ❑ B is usually squamous cell carcinoma (SCC)
- ❑ C usually occurs at the angle of the mouth
- ❑ D tends to metastasise to submandibular nodes
- ❑ E is radiosensitive

3.13 Medullary carcinoma of the thyroid

- ❑ A does not metastasise to cervical lymph nodes
- ❑ B is associated with multiple endocrine neoplasia (MEN) type I
- ❑ C may present as a solitary thyroid nodule
- ❑ D often contains amyloid
- ❑ E is treated by total thyroidectomy
- ❑ F is associated with calcitonin production
- ❑ G is associated with PTH production

3.14 In thyroid cancer

- ❑ A follicular carcinoma is usually treated by lobectomy alone
- ❑ B ^{131}I therapy has no role in the pre-operative management
- ❑ C treatment with high dose thyroxine is effective in reducing recurrence
- ❑ D chemotherapy can be effective in the treatment of recurrence
- ❑ E ^{131}I therapy can be used to treat local recurrence

3.15 The thyroglossal tract

- ❑ A usually persists as a small fistula
- ❑ B causes a small dimple in the tongue called the foramen caecum
- ❑ C may persist in parts as a thyroglossal cyst
- ❑ D is continuous with the pyramidal lobe of the thyroid
- ❑ E bifurcates around the hyoid bone

3.16 The differential diagnosis of a thyroglossal cyst includes

- ❑ A sub-hyoid bursa
- ❑ B thyroid swelling
- ❑ C epidermoid cyst
- ❑ D pharyngeal pouch
- ❑ E cystic hygroma

3.17 The following cause a simple goitre:

- ❑ A iodine deficiency
- ❑ B radiation
- ❑ C *E. coli*
- ❑ D diabetes mellitus
- ❑ E hypocalcaemia

3.18 The following are true about thyrotoxicosis:

- ❑ A many are caused by hot nodules
- ❑ B is often caused by immunoglobulins
- ❑ C patients have an increased appetite and weight
- ❑ D patients present with pretibial myxoedema
- ❑ E equal sex distribution

3.19 The following tumours are related to smoking:

- ❑ A squamous cell carcinoma of the cervix
- ❑ B acute myeloid leukaemia
- ❑ C transitional cell carcinoma of the bladder
- ❑ D non-Hodgkin's lymphoma
- ❑ E carcinoma of the larynx

3.20 The routine investigation of a thyroid lump includes

- ❑ A ultrasound
- ❑ B exercise ECG
- ❑ C isotope scan
- ❑ D CT scan neck
- ❑ E fine needle aspiration cytology
- ❑ F technetium-thallium subtraction scanning

3.21 The following are indicated in the investigation of a 30-year-old woman who has a lump in the right thyroid lobe and is euthyroid clinically:

- ❑ A electrocardiography
- ❑ B thyroid function tests
- ❑ C chest X-ray
- ❑ D ultrasound scan
- ❑ E fine needle aspiration cytology prior to imaging

3.22 Patients with a multi-nodular colloid goitre of the thyroid (MNCG)

- ❑ A may present with a cough
- ❑ B are usually hypothyroid
- ❑ C should always have a CT scan
- ❑ D should always have a radionucleotide scan
- ❑ E may have distended neck veins

3.23 Concerning tumours of the thyroid gland

- ❑ A all teratomas are malignant
- ❑ B follicular adenomas can be diagnosed on FNAC
- ❑ C papillary tumours spread via the lymphatic system
- ❑ D recurrent laryngeal nerve lesions are always a sign of malignancy
- ❑ E they may be familial

3.24 Thyroid disease

- ❑ A hot nodule
- ❑ B lymphoma
- ❑ C follicular adenoma
- ❑ D anaplastic carcinoma
- ❑ E follicular carcinoma

For each of the thyroid conditions above, select the most appropriate treatment or description.

1. radiotherapy and chemotherapy
2. resection and radiotherapy
3. Plummer's syndrome
4. hemi-thyroidectomy only
5. total thyroidectomy and radio iodine

3.25 Inguinal hernia in children

- ❑ A usually present with strangulation
- ❑ B frequently become irreducible in the first three months of life
- ❑ C require inguinal herniorrhaphy in most cases
- ❑ D should be repaired after one year of age
- ❑ E should be repaired without delivering the testicle into the wound
- ❑ F may contain ovary

3.26 The following are supplied by the recurrent laryngeal nerve:

- ❑ A all intrinsic laryngeal muscles
- ❑ B cricothyroid
- ❑ C sensation to subglottic region
- ❑ D sensory to the supraglottic region
- ❑ E sternothyroid

3.27 Following a thyroidectomy

- ❑ A the danger from bleeding is obviated by the use of large drains
- ❑ B complete recurrent laryngeal nerve division is more compromising than partial
- ❑ C respiratory distress may be due to pneumothorax
- ❑ D hypercalcaemia may occur due to manipulation of the parathyroid glands
- ❑ E the most common cause of respiratory distress is laryngeal oedema

3.28 Match the following

- ❑ A propylthiouracil
- ❑ B ^{131}I
- ❑ C carbimazole
- ❑ D dexamethasone
- ❑ E thyroxine

1. concentrated in toxic nodules
2. agranulocytosis
3. multinodular goitre
4. safe in breast feeding
5. thyroid crisis

3.29 The following are causes of respiratory distress following thyroidectomy:

- ❑ A unilateral recurrent laryngeal nerve section
- ❑ B aspiration
- ❑ C laryngeal oedema
- ❑ D hypocalcaemia
- ❑ E tracheomalacia

3.30 Excess parathyroid hormone

- ❑ A is associated with phalangeal exostosis
- ❑ B causes increased calcium absorption from the intestine
- ❑ C causes an increased production of 1,25 dihydrocholecalciferol
- ❑ D causes decreased excretion of potassium
- ❑ E causes increased laying down of woven bone

3.31 Concerning parathyroid glands

- ❑ A the lower glands originate from the 3rd branchial pouch
- ❑ B the glands are symmetrically distributed in 90%
- ❑ C the superior gland usually lies at the intersection of the RLN and the superior thyroid artery
- ❑ D the inferior gland may be found in the thyrothymic ligament
- ❑ E 3% of patients have an absent 4th gland

3.32 Hyperparathyroidism

- ☐ A primary hyperparathyroidism
- ☐ B secondary hyperparathyroidism
- ☐ C tertiary hyperparathyroidism
- ☐ D parathyroid hormone
- ☐ E hypoparathyroidism

For each of the points above, select the most appropriate answer from the list below.

1. osteoclast
2. normal serum calcium
3. adenoma
4. renal disease
5. thyroid surgery

3.33 The following are causes of hypercalcaemia:

- ☐ A Addison's disease
- ☐ B renal failure
- ☐ C diabetes mellitus
- ☐ D sarcoidosis
- ☐ E thyrotoxicosis

3.34 The following are features of hyperparathyroidism:

- ☐ A diarrhoea
- ☐ B peptic ulceration
- ☐ C renal calculi
- ☐ D brown tumours of bone
- ☐ E impaired glucose tolerance

3.35 The following are appropriate pre-operative localising techniques prior to parathyroidectomy:

- ❑ A none
- ❑ B ultrasound scan
- ❑ C sestaMIBI scan
- ❑ D venography
- ❑ E thallium/technetium scan

3.36 Congenital hypertrophic pyloric stenosis

- ❑ A presents with bilious vomiting following a test feed
- ❑ B has a positive family history in two-thirds of cases
- ❑ C typically presents at six months of age
- ❑ D may cause hypokalaemic alkalosis
- ❑ E is treated by Ramstedt's pyloromyotomy

3.37 The following are true concerning low calcium levels post parathyroidectomy:

- ❑ A hypocalcaemia on the first postoperative day indicates total parathyroid excision
- ❑ B asymptomatic corrected calcium level 2.0 mmol/l needs IV calcium treatment
- ❑ C absolute calcium levels are most useful
- ❑ D urgent treatment is needed for a symptomatic patient with a calcium level of 1.7 mmol/l with Calcichew
- ❑ E 1α cholecalciferol is shorter acting than calciferol

3.38 Pharyngeal web is associated with the following

- ❑ A megaloblastic anaemia
- ❑ B carcinoma
- ❑ C Plummer-Vinson syndrome
- ❑ D female sex
- ❑ E recurrent pneumonia

3.39 Pharyngeal pouch

- ❑ A is a pre-malignant condition
- ❑ B arises above thyropharyngeal membrane
- ❑ C may present with a mass in the anterior triangle of the neck
- ❑ D is associated with hiatus hernia
- ❑ E is a cause of Mendelsohn's syndrome

3.40 Tonsillectomy is indicated in the following:

- ❑ A two attacks of tonsillitis per year
- ❑ B respiratory obstruction
- ❑ C more than four attacks of tonsillitis per year
- ❑ D prophylactically before school age
- ❑ E at parents' request

3.41 Mesenteric adenitis

- ❑ A is frequently caused by a rotavirus
- ❑ B produces a high pyrexia
- ❑ C typically causes diffuse poorly localised pain
- ❑ D may give signs of peritonitis
- ❑ E produces a relative lymphocytosis

3.42 Laryngeal carcinoma

- ❑ A has an equal sex incidence
- ❑ B is most commonly supraglottic
- ❑ C usually presents with stridor
- ❑ D responds to radiotherapy
- ❑ E should be assessed by microlaryngoscopy in difficult cases

3.43 Complications following tonsillectomy include

- ❑ A bleeding that invariably responds to topical 1/10 000 adrenaline packs
- ❑ B complete dysphagia
- ❑ C secondary haemorrhage in 5%
- ❑ D secondary haemorrhage responding to antibiotics
- ❑ E quinsy

3.44 Concerning lumps in the parotid gland

- ❑ A 50% will be due to a parotid tumour
- ❑ B 90% of parotid tumours are adenomas
- ❑ C pleomorphic adenomas behave malignantly
- ❑ D they are likely to be malignant if facial nerve signs are present
- ❑ E they may be related to radiation exposure

3.45 In the neonate having surgery

- ❑ A nutrition is seldom a problem as nasogastric feeding can be started early in intestinal surgery
- ❑ B heat loss should be avoided by covering all exposed areas
- ❑ C the theatre should be kept at 30°C to avoid hypothermia
- ❑ D ventilation post-operatively should be used in abdominal operations via a cuffed ET tube
- ❑ E parenteral feeding is largely contraindicated in the neonate due to the inability of the liver to metabolise fatty acids

3.46 Oesophageal atresia

- ❑ A may be associated with cardiovascular anomalies
- ❑ B may be associated with urogenital anomalies
- ❑ C is usually associated with oligohydramnios
- ❑ D is suspected if cyanotic episodes occur during feeding
- ❑ E is diagnosed if the stomach is consistently empty on ultrasound scan

3.47 Concerning tumours of the thyroid gland

- ❑ A papillary carcinoma mainly affects women
- ❑ B follicular carcinoma can be diagnosed on FNAC
- ❑ C medullary carcinoma can be diagnosed on FNAC
- ❑ D anaplastic carcinoma can be treated with radiotherapy with good results
- ❑ E lymphoma confined to the thyroid gland should be treated with radiotherapy alone

3.48 The following are true of neonatal surgical conditions:

- ❑ A in gastroschisis there is no bowel herniation
- ❑ B there is a high incidence of associated anomalies with exomphalos
- ❑ C duodenal atresia is associated with polyhydramnios
- ❑ D duodenal atresia requires urgent duodenostomy
- ❑ E microcolon is associated with small bowel atresia

3.49 Intussusception

- ❑ A presents between the ages of 2 to 3 years
- ❑ B is ileocolic in the majority of cases
- ❑ C is usually found to have an anatomical cause
- ❑ D may be associated with a viral illness
- ❑ E may present with screaming attacks

4.1 Ileoanal pouch

- ❑ A should be offered to all patients who have had a panproctocolectomy
- ❑ B formation should be ideally covered by a defunctioning colostomy
- ❑ C is unlikely to be complicated by an enterocutaneous fistula
- ❑ D is commonly performed following total colectomy for Crohn's disease
- ❑ E produces approximately 4–7 defaecations per 24 hours

4.2 Cardinal features of abdominal obstruction include

- ❑ A constant abdominal pain
- ❑ B abdominal distension
- ❑ C vomiting
- ❑ D absolute constipation
- ❑ E pyrexia
- ❑ F coffee-ground vomiting
- ❑ G leucocytosis

4.3 The management of bowel obstruction includes

- ❑ A clear fluids only by mouth
- ❑ B NG tube if the patient has vomited recently
- ❑ C analgesia
- ❑ D immediate surgery in most patients
- ❑ E regular albumin

4.4 In large bowel obstruction

- ❑ A the small bowel is devoid of gas on a plain abdominal radiograph
- ❑ B the sigmoid colon is likely to perforate
- ❑ C sigmoid volvulus is more likely in the psychiatric population
- ❑ D early vomiting is a feature
- ❑ E the patient may pass stool normally on presentation

4.5 Calot's triangle

- ❑ A lies immediately lateral to the hepatic artery
- ❑ B is inferior to the visceral surface of the liver
- ❑ C is lateral to the common bile duct
- ❑ D contains the hepatic artery
- ❑ E contains a lymph node
- ❑ F may contain the right portal vein

4.6 The free border of the lesser omentum

- ❑ A is the aditus to the lesser sac
- ❑ B transmits the portal vein in front of the hepatic artery
- ❑ C the common bile duct is to the right of the hepatic artery
- ❑ D may have pressure applied to it in the Walker's manoeuvre
- ❑ E has four layers of peritoneum

4.7 A previously fit and well 58-year-old woman who has previously had a total abdominal hysterectomy and bilateral salpingo-oophorectomy presents with a two day history of small bowel obstruction. Probable causes include

- ❑ A obstructed femoral hernia
- ❑ B adhesions
- ❑ C small bowel atresia
- ❑ D obstructed incisional hernia
- ❑ E appendicitis
- ❑ F intussusception

4.8 Drugs used in *Helicobacter pylori* eradication include

- ❑ A metronidazole
- ❑ B lansoprazole
- ❑ C sucralfate
- ❑ D mebeverine
- ❑ E amoxycillin
- ❑ F mebendazole
- ❑ G pirenzepine

4.9 The immediate management of an 80-year-old man with an upper GI bleed includes

- ❑ A urinary catheter
- ❑ B upper GI endoscopy
- ❑ C proton pump inhibitor
- ❑ D central line
- ❑ E nasogastric tube
- ❑ F fluid replacement

4.10 Indications for surgery in upper gastrointestinal bleeds may include

- ❑ A patient > 55 years with three bleeds or more
- ❑ B patient > 60 years with two or more bleeds
- ❑ C initial haemoglobin level < 10 g/dl
- ❑ D transfusion requirement of six or more units
- ❑ E uncontrollable bleeding on endoscopy

4.11 A raised serum amylase may be present in the following:

- ❑ A perforated duodenal ulcer
- ❑ B lower lobe pneumonia
- ❑ C ruptured ectopic pregnancy
- ❑ D mesenteric infarction
- ❑ E biliary colic
- ❑ F post ERCP
- ❑ G Boerhaave's syndrome

4.12 The management of all patients with acute pancreatitis includes

- ❑ A insertion of urinary catheter
- ❑ B intravenous fluids only if shocked
- ❑ C avoidance of pethidine as it causes the sphincter of Oddi to contract
- ❑ D avoidance of antibiotics unless there is a proven area of necrosis
- ❑ E early transfer to high dependency unit
- ❑ F somatostatin
- ❑ G aprotinin

4.13 Removal of gallstones in a common bile duct may be achieved

- ❑ A percutaneously
- ❑ B at choledochoscopy
- ❑ C by ERCP
- ❑ D by lithotripsy
- ❑ E by gallstone dissolution agents
- ❑ F by open common bile duct exploration
- ❑ G by the Burhenne technique

4.14 Acute appendicitis

- ❑ A is common under the age of two years
- ❑ B results in raising of the white blood count
- ❑ C pain is usually preceded by vomiting
- ❑ D may present with diarrhoea
- ❑ E may have symptoms of a urinary tract infection
- ❑ F may be excluded with a positive MSU
- ❑ G is associated with a positive psoas stretch test
- ❑ H is associated with an Alvarado score of 8

4.15 The following are common causes of pyrexia one day post appendicectomy:

- ❑ A urinary tract infection
- ❑ B basal atelectasis
- ❑ C 'drip arm'
- ❑ D wound infection
- ❑ E ileus

4.16 The following are true of acute pancreatitis:

- ❑ A severity is proportional to the amylase rise
- ❑ B white blood count is a good prognostic indicator
- ❑ C it is most commonly caused by gallstones in UK
- ❑ D a patient may need insulin
- ❑ E a patient may need Creon (pancreatic supplements)

4.17 Anal fissure

- ❑ A results from a local collagen defect
- ❑ B causes classic pre-defaecatory pain
- ❑ C may be treated by topical agents
- ❑ D needs total internal anal sphincterotomy
- ❑ E is usually anterior in men
- ❑ F may be treated by glyceryl trinitrate cream
- ❑ G is associated with ulcerative colitis
- ❑ H is associated with colorectal carcinoma

4.18 Angiodysplasia

- ❑ A is a common cause of melaena
- ❑ B may cause massive bleeding
- ❑ C may be diagnosed by angiography
- ❑ D is usually situated at the sigmoid colon
- ❑ E may be treated endoscopically

4.19 Perianal abscess

- ❑ A is unusual in the inter-sphincteric plane
- ❑ B may cause fistulae
- ❑ C obeys Goodsall's Law
- ❑ D may be drained internally
- ❑ E may need MRI for assessment

4.20 Pancreatic trauma

- ❑ A occurs in approximately 10% of major abdominal injuries
- ❑ B may be associated with duodenal injury
- ❑ C most commonly occurs in the pancreatic body
- ❑ D produces a high concentration of amylase in diagnostic peritoneal lavage fluid which is pathognomic
- ❑ E should be investigated by ERCP and CT

4.21 Carcinoma of the gall bladder

- ❑ A is the most common malignancy of the biliary tract
- ❑ B is usually diagnosed by ultrasound
- ❑ C is strongly associated with gallstones
- ❑ D is associated with gall bladder polyps
- ❑ E has a good response to adjuvant chemotherapy

4.22 Umbilical hernia

- ❑ A is four times more common in Afro-Caribbean than in Caucasian children
- ❑ B defect usually closes by four years of age
- ❑ C in adults frequently contains bowel
- ❑ D may be closed using a Mayo repair
- ❑ E is usually repaired using a mesh
- ❑ F is common in chronic obstructive pulmonary disease

4.23 Obturator hernia

- ❑ A is commoner in men
- ❑ B presents with a lump in the upper inner aspect of the thigh
- ❑ C commonly causes knee pain
- ❑ D is most frequently found at laparotomy
- ❑ E is repaired by direct apposition of the margins of the defect

4.24 After total colectomy for ulcerative colitis the following options are satisfactory for different patients

- ❑ A Kock pouch
- ❑ B ileorectal anastomosis
- ❑ C ileal pouch anal anastomosis
- ❑ D end ileostomy
- ❑ E mucous fistula

4.25 Proctitis may be caused by the following:

- ❑ A *chlamydia trachomatis*
- ❑ B *neisseria gonorrhoea*
- ❑ C herpes simplex
- ❑ D *ascaris lumbricoides*
- ❑ E radiotherapy

4.26 Haemorrhoids

- ❑ A are obstructed anal veins
- ❑ B may deteriorate with cirrhosis
- ❑ C may resolve with diet
- ❑ D may be treated by band ligation
- ❑ E may be treated with submucosal injection of 80% phenol

4.27 With regard to carcinoma of the oesophagus

- ❑ A the patient does not lose weight on presentation
- ❑ B the patient presents with equal dysphagia for solids and liquids
- ❑ C it is the most common in the middle third of the oesophagus
- ❑ D a chest X-ray is useful but not essential
- ❑ E it is usually an adenocarcinoma in the Western world

4.28 The following are associated with right upper qua…

- ❑ A sickle cell disease
- ❑ B pelvic inflammatory disease
- ❑ C inguinal hernia
- ❑ D appendicitis
- ❑ E peptic ulcer

4.29 Epigastric pain may be caused by

- ❑ A peptic ulcer
- ❑ B diverticular disease
- ❑ C myocardial infarction
- ❑ D diabetes mellitus
- ❑ E gastro-oesphageal reflux
- ❑ F pericarditis

4.30 Diarrhoea may be related to

- ❑ A chronic pancreatitis
- ❑ B Zollinger-Ellison syndrome
- ❑ C gastric surgery
- ❑ D inflammatory bowel disease
- ❑ E codeine abuse
- ❑ F colonic resection

4.31 With regard to rectal cancer

- ❑ A the most important margins at AP excision are the proximal ones
- ❑ B it usually presents with iron deficiency anaemia
- ❑ C it may present with diarrhoea
- ❑ D it may be confused with inflammatory bowel disease
- ❑ E pre-operative radiotherapy has no benefit

4.32 Features of ulcerative colitis include the following:

- ❑ A ileum always spared
- ❑ B transmural inflammation
- ❑ C increased risk of malignancy
- ❑ D cobble stone mucosa on barium enema
- ❑ E commonly presents with bloody diarrhoea
- ❑ F granuloma formation

4.33 The following should be considered before operating on a jaundiced patient:

- ❑ A fluid restriction
- ❑ B mannitol infusion
- ❑ C chest physiotherapy
- ❑ D antibiotics
- ❑ E intravenous heparin

4.34 Liver function may be assessed by the following:

- ❑ A serum bilirubin
- ❑ B coagulation assay
- ❑ C detoxification of sulphonylureas
- ❑ D albumin
- ❑ E creatinine kinase titres

4.35 Gallstones impacted in the common bile duct may be treated by the following:

- ❑ A endoscopic retrograde cholangio-pancreatography
- ❑ B cholecystostomy
- ❑ C hepatico-docho-jejunostomy
- ❑ D percutaneous transhepatic cholangiography
- ❑ E ursodeoxycholic acid

4.36 A tender right iliac fossa in a 30-year-old man may be due to

❑ A acute appendicitis
❑ B cholecystitis
❑ C mittleschmerz
❑ D duodenal ulcer
❑ E pancreatitis

4.37 Right iliac fossa pain may be related to

❑ A ovarian disease
❑ B Crohn's disease
❑ C tuberculosis
❑ D hip fracture
❑ E lymphoma
❑ F colonic diverticula

4.38 Risk factors for peptic ulcer disease include

❑ A blood group
❑ B alcohol
❑ C *Helicobacter pylori*
❑ D prednisolone
❑ E metformin

4.39 Posterior relations of the stomach include

❑ A right kidney
❑ B head of the pancreas
❑ C left psoas muscle
❑ D left adrenal gland
❑ E left hemidiaphragm

4.40 Immediate branches of the coeliac artery include

- ❑ A superior mesenteric artery
- ❑ B gastrojejunal artery
- ❑ C hepatic artery
- ❑ D splenic artery
- ❑ E short gastric arteries
- ❑ F cystic artery

4.41 The following are causes of obstructive jaundice:

- ❑ A intra-vascular haemolysis
- ❑ B carcinoma of the head of the pancreas
- ❑ C gallstones confined to the gall bladder fundus
- ❑ D colonic cancer
- ❑ E cholangiocarcinoma
- ❑ F Mirizzi syndrome

4.42 The following are true for acholuric jaundice:

- ❑ A dark urine
- ❑ B intra-vascular haemolysis
- ❑ C caused by carcinoma of the head of the pancreas
- ❑ D associated with a normal alkaline phosphatase level
- ❑ E associated with increased transaminases

4.43 Hepatocellular jaundice causes

- ❑ A steatorrhoea
- ❑ B dark urine
- ❑ C grossly elevated alkaline phosphatase levels
- ❑ D grossly elevated transaminase levels
- ❑ E a mixed picture of a raised conjugated and unconjugated bilirubin

4.44 The following may present with indigestion:

- ❑ A colonic carcinoma
- ❑ B gallstones
- ❑ C coronary atherosclerosis
- ❑ D Colles' fracture
- ❑ E mesenteric angina

4.45 The following are true of visceral pain:

- ❑ A is caused by the irritation of the pleura or peritoneum
- ❑ B is caused by the activation of stretch receptors
- ❑ C is usually well localised
- ❑ D often radiates
- ❑ E is usually unhelpful in making a diagnosis

4.46 Biliary colic

- ❑ A causes right upper quadrant pain
- ❑ B causes vomiting
- ❑ C leads to a raised white blood count
- ❑ D is usually associated with a raised temperature
- ❑ E lasts for about 4 to 10 minutes in duration

4.47 The blood supply of the oesophagus is from the following:

- ❑ A left hepatic artery
- ❑ B left inferior phrenic artery
- ❑ C superior thyroid artery
- ❑ D bronchial artery
- ❑ E left gastric artery

4.48 Dysphagia may be associated with the following:

❑ A congenital syndromes
❑ B anaemia
❑ C asthma-like symptoms
❑ D aortic aneurysm
❑ E mitral stenosis

4.49 Relations of the intra-thoracic oesophagus include

❑ A trachea
❑ B left lobe of the liver
❑ C accessory hemiazygous vein
❑ D pericardium
❑ E right main bronchus
❑ F inferior vena cava

4.50 The following are true about abdominal incisions:

❑ A midline incisions are associated with more blood loss than paramedian
❑ B transverse incisions are associated with fewer respiratory complications
❑ C transverse incisions are quick to make
❑ D paramedian incisions give good access
❑ E midline incisions give the best cosmetic result

4.51 Ileostomy

❑ A is always permanent
❑ B may lead to hypokalaemia
❑ C may cause a chronic microcytic anaemia
❑ D should be flush with the vein
❑ E may lead to right upper quadrant pain

4.52 Caecostomy

- ❑ A is never performed in modern surgical practice
- ❑ B may be useful to decompress the colon
- ❑ C is useful to decompress the ileum
- ❑ D is used for feeding
- ❑ E inadequately diverts the faecal stream

4.53 The following are true about truncal vagotomy:

- ❑ A it preserves the pyloric fibres
- ❑ B it may cause dumping
- ❑ C it may cause constipation
- ❑ D it may cause gastritis
- ❑ E it may cause gastric stasis

4.54 In Zollinger-Ellison syndrome the following are true:

- ❑ A gastrin levels are reduced
- ❑ B gastrin levels fall on secretin administration
- ❑ C it is associated with small bowel hamartomata
- ❑ D it is the only cause of raised gastrin levels
- ❑ E it always requires surgery

4.55 Hepatomegaly occurs in the following:

- ❑ A cirrhosis
- ❑ B carcinoma of the lung
- ❑ C hepatitis
- ❑ D left ventricular failure
- ❑ E malaria

4.56 In femoral herniae

- ❑ A the vein is medial to the artery
- ❑ B the hernia is between the artery and vein
- ❑ C the hernia is easily palpable below and lateral to the pubic tubercle
- ❑ D obstruction is rarely caused
- ❑ E more patients are women than men

4.57 Herniae

- ❑ A associated with pain indicate obstruction
- ❑ B found with small bowel are more often a left sided inguinal hernia
- ❑ C may be strangulated if tender, irreducible and associated with a cough impulse
- ❑ D are always palpable
- ❑ E are Littre's herniae if behind the rectus sheath

4.58 A Kocher's incision

- ❑ A divides Colles' fascia
- ❑ B divides only the anterior rectus sheath, the posterior being deficient
- ❑ C divides external oblique
- ❑ D involves the area innervated by T10 nerve root
- ❑ E divides the fascia transversalis
- ❑ F divides the rectus abdominis muscle

4.59 A perforated duodenal ulcer

- ❑ A may mimic acute appendicitis
- ❑ B needs oversewing and truncal vagotomy
- ❑ C needs biopsy to exclude malignancy
- ❑ D should have four quadrant drains inserted after a washout
- ❑ E is adequately treated by an oversew patch and washout only

4.60 The following are true of acute cholecystitis:

- ❑ A early cholecystectomy is a suitable treatment
- ❑ B surgery should be avoided with empyema and peritonism
- ❑ C cholecystectomy should be delayed for eight weeks after the presentation
- ❑ D empyema may be treated by cholecystostomy
- ❑ E it usually resolves on conservative treatment

4.61 Charcot's triad consists of

- ❑ A fever
- ❑ B leucocytosis
- ❑ C rigors
- ❑ D gallstones
- ❑ E jaundice
- ❑ F diverticular disease
- ❑ G elevated serum amylase

4.62 The lienorenal ligament contains the following:

- ❑ A splenic artery
- ❑ B renal artery
- ❑ C tail of the pancreas
- ❑ D portal vein
- ❑ E splenic vein
- ❑ F the left adrenal gland

4.63 Gastric acid secretion

- ❑ A occurs in four phases
- ❑ B is increased by histamine
- ❑ C is reduced by acetylcholine
- ❑ D is reduced by prostaglandins
- ❑ E is increased by renin

4.64 Complications of a chronic duodenal ulcer include

- ❑ A anaemia
- ❑ B gastric outlet obstruction
- ❑ C jaundice
- ❑ D perforation
- ❑ E symptoms of hypocalcaemia

4.65 Pancreatic pseudocysts

- ❑ A may resolve spontaneously
- ❑ B are more common in alcoholic pancreatitis
- ❑ C should be drained early
- ❑ D may be drained endoscopically
- ❑ E are preferably drained externally rather than internally
- ❑ F occur in the body of the pancreas

4.66 A 70-year-old man presents with sudden onset severe constant upper abdominal pain; causes include

- ❑ A myocardial infarction
- ❑ B perforated duodenal ulcer
- ❑ C mesenteric ischaemia
- ❑ D small bowel obstruction
- ❑ E leaking abdominal aortic aneurysm
- ❑ F pericarditis

4.67 Immediate routine investigations of a patient who presents as an emergency with epigastric pain include

- ❑ A full blood count
- ❑ B abdominal ultrasound
- ❑ C erect chest X-ray
- ❑ D amylase
- ❑ E liver function tests

4.68 Oesophageal varices

- ❑ A have an associated mortality of 1% if from an extrahepatic block in the absence of liver disease
- ❑ B are portosystemic anastamoses
- ❑ C may be treated with intra vasal sclerosant
- ❑ D may be treated by band ligation
- ❑ E may be treated by paravasal sclerosant injection

4.69 The following are used for Child's classification of portal hypertension:

- ❑ A bilirubin
- ❑ B ascites
- ❑ C portal pressure (cm H_2O)
- ❑ D prothrombin time
- ❑ E amylase
- ❑ F presence of oesophageal varices

4.70 Gastric erosions may

- ❑ A be caused by NSAIDs
- ❑ B be caused by burns
- ❑ C be diagnosed by barium meal
- ❑ D be treated by sucralfate
- ❑ E give similar symptoms to an ulcer

4.71 Barrett's oesophagus

- ❑ A is a pre-malignant condition
- ❑ B is rarely seen at endoscopy
- ❑ C is associated with a 30-fold increased risk of cancer
- ❑ D may be associated with benign strictures
- ❑ E may be associated with refractory ulcers

4.72 Achalasia

- ❑ A is always diagnosed on a barium swallow
- ❑ B shows characteristic waves in the oesophagus
- ❑ C leads to a progressive dysphagia, solids affected first
- ❑ D responds well to dilatation
- ❑ E may indicate Keller's operation

4.73 With regard to perforation of the oesophagus

- ❑ A it may follow a large vomit
- ❑ B it may be treated conservatively
- ❑ C delayed presentation should be treated surgically
- ❑ D the degree of contamination is not relevant to the treatment choice
- ❑ E enteral feeding should be started immediately

4.74 The following is true for gastro-oesophageal reflux disease (GORD):

- ❑ A patients should have an ECG if the diagnosis is uncertain
- ❑ B it may respond to conservative treatments
- ❑ C it always responds to proton pump inhibitors
- ❑ D patients may have a normal barium swallow
- ❑ E patients may have symptoms on 40 mg omeprazole daily
- ❑ F it is usually treated by laparoscopic fundoplication

4.75 Proton pump inhibitors (PPIs)

- ❑ A have proven safe for long term use
- ❑ B may cause gastritis
- ❑ C are the first line treatment for GORD
- ❑ D may cause a dry cough
- ❑ E often cause diarrhoea leading to failure of compliance

4.76 The following are true of oesophagitis:

- ❑ A grade 4 disease has a normal barium swallow
- ❑ B Barrett's oesophagus leads to squamous carcinoma
- ❑ C benign strictures are readily differentiated clinically from malignant ones
- ❑ D it may be due to alkaline reflux
- ❑ E it may mimic cardiac pain

4.77 Herniae

- ❑ A the most common type of hernia in female adults is femoral
- ❑ B direct inguinal herniae often strangulate
- ❑ C inguinal herniae are more common on the right
- ❑ D infant inguinal herniae have a ratio male:female 3:2
- ❑ E direct inguinal herniae are common in women

4.78 Herniae

- ❑ A are usually diagnosed by a herniogram
- ❑ B are usually diagnosed by ultrasound
- ❑ C may strangulate without obstruction
- ❑ D are easily distinguished direct from indirect clinically by their relation to the internal ring
- ❑ E may be the presenting symptom of malignancy

4.79 The following are true about the inguinal canal:

- ❑ A the deep ring is at the mid inguinal point
- ❑ B it transmits the ilio-inguinal nerve
- ❑ C the fascia transversalis forms the posterior wall
- ❑ D it is empty in women
- ❑ E it is long and thin in children

4.80 The characteristic features of ulcerative colitis include

- ❑ A crypt abscesses
- ❑ B pseudopolyps
- ❑ C goblet cells
- ❑ D transmural inflammation
- ❑ E superficial ulceration
- ❑ F granulomata
- ❑ G deeply fissured ulcers

4.81 Epigastric hernia

- ❑ A is most common in children
- ❑ B affects men 3 times more frequently than women
- ❑ C is rarely multiple
- ❑ D usually contains omentum
- ❑ E normally requires repair with prolene mesh

4.82 Acute mesenteric ischaemia

- ❑ A is caused by a superior mesenteric embolus in up to 50% cases
- ❑ B is associated with congestive cardiac failure
- ❑ C leads to severe haemoconcentration
- ❑ D rarely produces hypovolaemic shock
- ❑ E always produces marked abdominal signs
- ❑ F is associated with increased plasma lactate levels

4.83 Paraoesophageal hiatus hernia

- ❑ A has a higher prevalence of dysphagia compared with sliding hiatus hernia
- ❑ B has a lower incidence of post-prandial fullness compared with sliding hiatus hernia
- ❑ C may present with haematemesis in 1/3 of cases
- ❑ D is associated with recurrent pneumonia
- ❑ E is associated with gastric volvulus
- ❑ F should be repaired electively when found

4.84 Meckel's diverticulum

- ❑ A is usually lined by gastric mucosa
- ❑ B can be found in an inguinal hernia
- ❑ C is inherited
- ❑ D may contain heterotopic pancreatic tissue
- ❑ E is most commonly complicated by inflammation
- ❑ F causes intussusception
- ❑ G should be removed if found incidentally

4.85 Diverticulosis of the small bowel

- ❑ A is most common in the ileum
- ❑ B is rare
- ❑ C is always found on the mesenteric border
- ❑ D is usually symptomless
- ❑ E can give rise to vitamin B_{12} deficiency

4.86 Acute diverticulitis of the colon

- ❑ A produces bowel wall thickening which may be seen on CT
- ❑ B may be accurately diagnosed by gastrografin enema
- ❑ C settles with iv antibiotics alone in 50% of cases
- ❑ D may be treated by colectomy and primary anastomosis
- ❑ E when treated medically recurs in 70% cases
- ❑ F is a premalignant disease

4.87 Bile duct injury following laparoscopic cholecystectomy

- ❑ A occurs in 3% cases
- ❑ B typically presents with right upper quadrant inflammation and irritation
- ❑ C may lead to subsequent biliary stricturing
- ❑ D is best investigated by repeat laparoscopy
- ❑ E can be reduced if diathermy is avoided near the biliary ducts
- ❑ F is prevented by intraoperative cholangiography

4.88 Carcinoid tumour of the appendix

- ❑ A may be associated with carcinoid of the ileum
- ❑ B is found at the base in 25% cases
- ❑ C usually affects children in their teens
- ❑ D is found incidentally on routine histology in most cases
- ❑ E commonly gives rise to carcinoid syndrome

4.89 Pseudomembranous colitis

- ❑ A is commonly severe and life-threatening
- ❑ B may be caused by intravenous cefuroxime
- ❑ C is treated with intravenous vancomycin
- ❑ D produces a characteristic red-brown membrane
- ❑ E may be diagnosed by demonstration of toxin in the faeces

4.90 Acute cholecystitis

- ❑ A may occur in the absence of gallstones
- ❑ B develops primarily as a result of bacterial infection
- ❑ C usually produces a palpable mass
- ❑ D may be accurately diagnosed by ultrasound in over 95% cases
- ❑ E causes absence of gall bladder labelling in 99 mTc HIDA scan
- ❑ F may cause jaundice
- ❑ G is usually an indication for urgent cholecystectomy

4.91 Acute pancreatitis

- ❑ A is a recognised complication following gastrectomy
- ❑ B is caused by gallstones in 80% cases
- ❑ C is associated with cardiopulmonary bypass
- ❑ D decreases pulmonary compliance
- ❑ E gives rise to pseudocysts in 30% cases

4.92 Poor prognostic factors in acute pancreatitis include

- ❑ A amylase > 2000 iu/l
- ❑ B $PaO_2 < 8$ kPa
- ❑ C $PaCO_2 > 5$ kPa
- ❑ D WBC > 20×10^9/l
- ❑ E LDH > 600 iu/l

4.93 Colonic carcinoma

- ❑ A is more common following cholecystectomy
- ❑ B has a 1 in 50 risk of death in Western populations
- ❑ C has a 1 in 10 risk of death in patients with a single relative with colorectal cancer
- ❑ D is synchronous in 20% cases
- ❑ E presents with pulmonary metastases in 10% cases

4.94 Splenic flexure colonic carcinoma

- ❑ A has a high local recurrence rate
- ❑ B has a poor survival rate regardless of stage and presentation
- ❑ C may be treated by extended right hemicolectomy
- ❑ D may be treated by left hemicolectomy

4.95 Anal cancer

- ❑ A usually arises from anal glands
- ❑ B is associated with a five-fold increased risk with a history of genital warts
- ❑ C may present with inguinal lymph node involvement in up to 30% cases
- ❑ D most commonly presents with a lump
- ❑ E should ideally be examined under anaesthesia

4.96 Ulcerative colitis

- ❑ A most commonly presents with proctitis
- ❑ B is characterised in 70% cases by granuloma formation
- ❑ C only affects the mucosal layer
- ❑ D affects the splenic flexure in 20% cases
- ❑ E is associated with primary sclerosing cholangitis

4.97 Acute pseudocysts of the pancreas

- ❑ A have a cyst wall composed of fibrous and granulation tissue
- ❑ B may be found in the mediastinum
- ❑ C are usually found in the lesser sac
- ❑ D do not occur following trauma
- ❑ E cause a persistently raised amylase in 50% cases

4.98 Chronic pancreatitis

- ❑ A is usually the result of gallstones
- ❑ B is more common in men
- ❑ C may be due to pancreas divisum
- ❑ D may be inherited
- ❑ E produces a 'chain of lakes' appearance on ERCP

4.99 In the management of pain due to chronic pancreatitis

- ❑ A cessation of all alcohol intake is important
- ❑ B morphine sulphate tablets should be commenced immediately
- ❑ C sphincterotomy of the sphincter of Oddi may be helpful
- ❑ D coeliac ganglia destruction may be helpful
- ❑ E pancreaticojejunostomy is useful if the ducts are dilated

4.100 Zollinger-Ellison syndrome

- ❑ A usually presents at 50 years of age
- ❑ B should be suspected if a peptic ulcer is refractory to treatment
- ❑ C patients typically have ulcers in unusual locations
- ❑ D is frequently caused by a benign granuloma
- ❑ E is not amenable to medical management
- ❑ F can be assessed using an octreotide scan

4.101 Periampullary pancreatic carcinoma

- ❑ A is found at the ampulla of Vater in 30% of cases
- ❑ B is histologically most commonly a ductal adenocarcinoma
- ❑ C has no known risk factors
- ❑ D is associated with familial adenomatous polyposis
- ❑ E may cause elevation of CA 19–9

4.102 Pancreatic pseudocysts

- ❑ A occur only after acute pancreatitis
- ❑ B are likely to resolve spontaneously if < 6 cm in diameter
- ❑ C mostly communicate with a major pancreatic duct
- ❑ D are associated with high mortality in cases of spontaneous rupture
- ❑ E are successfully drained by a single percutaneous aspiration
- ❑ F are collections of fluid in a cyst in the pancreas

4.103 The spleen

- ❑ A lies deep to the 9, 10, 11th ribs
- ❑ B is suspended partly by the gastrosplenic ligament containing the gastroepiploic vessels
- ❑ C is contained in a capsule approximately 1 cm thick
- ❑ D removes Howell-Jolly bodies from the circulation
- ❑ E is the only site of red cell destruction

SYSTEM MODULE E: URINARY SYSTEM AND RENAL TRANSPLANTATION

5.1 The indications for a transurethral resection of prostate (TURP) include

- ❑ A outflow obstruction
- ❑ B recurrent UTIs
- ❑ C failed trial without catheter
- ❑ D first episode of acute urinary retention
- ❑ E frequent nocturia with outflow obstruction from an enlarged prostate

5.2 The following may present as prostatism:

- ❑ A congenital urethral valves
- ❑ B spinal injury
- ❑ C tricyclic antidepressants
- ❑ D diverticular disease
- ❑ E Parkinson's disease

5.3 Blood in the urine

- ❑ A may be normal
- ❑ B is urethral in origin if it precedes micturition
- ❑ C is renal in origin at the end of voiding
- ❑ D is of no significance if the patient is on anticoagulants
- ❑ E may not be visible to the naked eye

5.4 With regard to renal function

- ❑ A urea is a good indicator
- ❑ B creatinine production is related to muscle mass
- ❑ C creatinine is excreted by glomerular filtration and tubular secretion
- ❑ D failure may be assessed with arterial blood gases
- ❑ E clearance may be measured using EDTA

5.5 Renal adenocarcinoma

❑ A most commonly presents in men in their late 30s
❑ B may produce hypercalcaemia
❑ C patients often have metastases at time of presentation
❑ D often produces abnormal renal function
❑ E is associated with tuberose sclerosis

5.6 Wilms' tumour (nephroblastoma)

❑ A most commonly presents before five years of age
❑ B is associated with genitourinary tract abnormalities
❑ C invariably produces haematuria
❑ D commonly metastasises to the lung
❑ E is relatively resistant to radiotherapy

5.7 Bladder cancer

❑ A has an equal male to female incidence ratio
❑ B produces painless haematuria in 85% cases
❑ C usually arises in the anterior wall of the bladder
❑ D caused by stones is usually adenocarcinoma in origin
❑ E may be caused by schistosomiasis

5.8 Urothelial transitional cell carcinoma (TCC)

❑ A is more common in men
❑ B has increased incidence among rubber workers
❑ C affects the bladder in 95% of cases
❑ D usually presents with haematuria
❑ E frequently presents with polycythaemia
❑ F may be treated by intravesical erythromycin
❑ G is radio-resistant
❑ H is commonly multicentric

5.9 Horseshoe kidney

- ❑ A is more common in women
- ❑ B usually has a standard blood supply
- ❑ C is more prone to infection
- ❑ D is more prone to trauma
- ❑ E may complicate aortic aneurysm repair

5.10 Renal cysts

- ❑ A are usually benign
- ❑ B are common in the over 70s
- ❑ C pain or bleeding into a renal cyst are of no significance
- ❑ D should not be aspirated to prevent retroperitoneal fibrosis
- ❑ E may be due to infection

5.11 Ureteric injury

- ❑ A is most commonly due to iatrogenic damage
- ❑ B may result in a ureterovaginal fistula
- ❑ C should always be managed by primary direct repair
- ❑ D may be repaired in the lower 1/3 of the ureter by a Brooke bladder flap
- ❑ E may be repaired with 5′0′ prolene sutures

5.12 In genito-urinary tract trauma

- ❑ A an absent nephrogram on IVU may suggest renal pedicle avulsion
- ❑ B the amount of haematuria correlates well with the severity of injury
- ❑ C a high riding prostate is a contraindication to urethral catheterisation
- ❑ D retrograde ureteric catheterisation is useful in assessing state of injury
- ❑ E the retroperitoneal haematoma may cause a paralytic ileus

5.13 Prostatic adenocarcinoma

- ❑ A has lifetime risk of approximately 2%
- ❑ B usually arises in the peripheral zone of the gland
- ❑ C is a recognised cause of haematuria
- ❑ D bony secondaries usually appear as lytic lesions on plain X-rays
- ❑ E is radio-resistant
- ❑ F is sensitive to androgen deprivation

5.14 Ovarian cancer

- ❑ A peak incidence occurs during the 5th and 6th decades
- ❑ B risk is increased by early menopause
- ❑ C often causes a rise in serum alpha-fetoprotein
- ❑ D may present with bowel obstruction
- ❑ E mainstay of management is radiotherapy

5.15 Testicular neoplasms

- ❑ A are most common in men under 40
- ❑ B can usually be safely biopsied by fine needle aspiration
- ❑ C have an overall survival of > 80% due to surgery
- ❑ D are commoner in the contralateral side in patients having orchidopexy
- ❑ E are usually excised through a transverse scrotal incision

5.16 The bladder

- ❑ A is covered entirely by peritoneum
- ❑ B is separated from the rectum by Denonvillier's fascia
- ❑ C is relatively fixed at the trigone
- ❑ D has the ureters entering near its lateral walls
- ❑ E receives its blood supply from a branch of the external iliac artery

5.17 Prostate carcinoma

- ❑ A is rare below the age of 50 years
- ❑ B typically arises in the periphery of the prostate
- ❑ C usually metastasises to the thoracic spine
- ❑ D when confined within the prostate capsule is defined as T3
- ❑ E most frequently presents with symptoms of bladder outflow obstruction

5.18 Polycystic renal disease

- ❑ A may be an autosomal recessive disorder
- ❑ B may present as an adult or an infantile form
- ❑ C may be an autosomal dominant disease
- ❑ D rarely causes renal failure
- ❑ E is an absolute indication for transplant

5.19 With regard to ureteric duplication

- ❑ A the lower ureter enters the bladder inferiorly
- ❑ B reflux is uncommon
- ❑ C the lower pole ureter is most likely to reflux
- ❑ D it is commonly bilateral
- ❑ E UTIs are common

5.20 With regard to a plain abdominal X-ray renal trauma is likely if

- ❑ A the psoas shadow is outlined more clearly
- ❑ B there are fractured ribs 10, 11, 12
- ❑ C there is scoliosis to the injured side
- ❑ D Riggler's sign is present
- ❑ E there are fractures of transverse process of T5

5.21 The following are features of acute pyelonephritis:

- ❑ A rigors
- ❑ B loin tenderness
- ❑ C pyrexia
- ❑ D gross haematuria
- ❑ E renal failure

5.22 The following drugs may be useful in the treatment of metastatic prostate carcinoma:

- ❑ A cyproterone
- ❑ B flutamide
- ❑ C goserelin
- ❑ D tamoxifen
- ❑ E bumetanide
- ❑ F finasteride
- ❑ G leuprorelin
- ❑ H aminoglutethimide

5.23 Testicular seminoma is

- ❑ A a recognised cause of gynaecomastia
- ❑ B usually diagnosed by needle biopsy
- ❑ C radio resistant
- ❑ D resistant to chemotherapy
- ❑ E associated with disease free survival of 99% for stage I disease

5.24 Testicular seminoma

- ❑ A presents with a lump in the scrotum in 80% cases
- ❑ B produces cannon ball metastases in the lungs
- ❑ C may secrete beta hCG
- ❑ D is very radio-sensitive
- ❑ E may present with a history of trauma

5.25 Carcinoma of the penis

- ❑ A usually presents early
- ❑ B involves the inguinal lymph nodes in 50% cases at presentation
- ❑ C is relatively radio-resistant
- ❑ D has an overall poor long term survival in the absence of lymphadenopathy

5.26 Priapism

- ❑ A is associated with sickle cell anaemia
- ❑ B usually produces an engorged corpus spongiosum
- ❑ C may be helped by injection of metaraminol
- ❑ D may be treated by embolisation of the pudendal vessels
- ❑ E may be treated by a corporasaphenous shunt
- ❑ F is associated with chronic lymphatic leukaemia
- ❑ G is associated with porphyria

5.27 Match the following

- ❑ A renal carbuncle
- ❑ B acute pyelonephritis
- ❑ C chronic pyelonephritis
- ❑ D pyonephrosis
- ❑ E perinephric abscess

Match the treatments/sequelae below to the appropriate renal pathology above.

1. hypertension
2. nephrostomy
3. antibiotics
4. incision and drainage
5. ultrasound drainage

5.28 The following are features of renal TB:

- ❑ A ureteric stricture
- ❑ B peak incidence age 25 years
- ❑ C dysuria
- ❑ D frequency

5.29 Ureteric obstruction may occur from the following:

- ❑ A colitis
- ❑ B retroperitoneal fibrosis
- ❑ C arterial disease
- ❑ D pancreatitis
- ❑ E lymphoma

5.30 With regard to renal tract calculi

- ❑ A the incidence is increasing
- ❑ B they are more common in horseshoe kidney
- ❑ C the majority are mixed phosphate in content
- ❑ D they are more common in vegetarians
- ❑ E they are more common in the presence of reflux

5.31 Undescended testis

- ❑ A is present in 40% full term male births
- ❑ B is bilateral in 20% cases
- ❑ C is usually found at the base of the penis
- ❑ D has a higher rate of torsion
- ❑ E is at a higher risk of carcinomatous change despite orchidopexy

5.32 Torsion of the testis

- ❑ A may present with lower abdominal pain
- ❑ B is predisposed by a short testicular mesorchium
- ❑ C may be accurately diagnosed by ultrasound
- ❑ D may mimic an inflammatory testicular tumour
- ❑ E may be repaired using the Jaboulay technique

5.33 Nephroblastoma

- ❑ A is associated with hemihypertrophy
- ❑ B is bilateral 25%
- ❑ C presents with failure to thrive
- ❑ D presents with sterile pyuria
- ❑ E presents with haematuria

5.34 Renal cell carcinoma

- ❑ A primary tumours are usually clear cell tumours
- ❑ B is more common in women
- ❑ C is associated with aromatic hydrocarbons
- ❑ D is associated with asbestos
- ❑ E predominantly spreads via lymphatics

5.35 Renal transplant

- ❑ A acute rejection
- ❑ B hyperacute rejection
- ❑ C chronic rejection
- ❑ D blood group mismatch

Match the following concerning transplantation.

1. humoral system
2. cellular immunity
3. haemolysis
4. pre-sensitisation

5.36 Idiopathic scrotal oedema

- ❑ A usually affects children between 8–12 years of age
- ❑ B is usually painful
- ❑ C may affect the groin and thighs
- ❑ D is diagnosed by ultrasound
- ❑ E resolves without treatment in a few days

5.37 Acute epididymitis

- ❑ A is rare before puberty
- ❑ B has no identifying underlying cause in 50% of cases
- ❑ C rarely causes a secondary hydrocele
- ❑ D with urethral discharge is most commonly due to *Chlamydia*
- ❑ E may lead to testicular atrophy

5.38 The following are in keeping with acute renal failure:

- ❑ A low volume of urine
- ❑ B specific gravity 1030
- ❑ C urinary sodium 15 mmol/l
- ❑ D urinary urea 160 mmol/l
- ❑ E osmolarity 300 mmol/kg water

5.39 The following may complicate a urethral stricture:

- ❑ A fistulae
- ❑ B rectal prolapse
- ❑ C hyperparathyroidism
- ❑ D periurethral abscess
- ❑ E renal failure

5.40 Hypospadias

- ❑ A is not normally associated with a chordee
- ❑ B most commonly occurs at the coronal or glandular meatus
- ❑ C should be corrected operatively at 2–3 years of age
- ❑ D correction should aim to site the meatus at the tip of the penis
- ❑ E is a rare abnormality of penile development

5.41 Bladder calculi

- ❑ A usually arise from calculi passed down the ureter
- ❑ B occur in bladder diverticula
- ❑ C classically present with lower abdominal pain
- ❑ D are commonly associated with UTI
- ❑ E may lead to transitional cell carcinoma in long standing cases

5.42 The following are sites of ectopic testes:

- ❑ A deep inguinal ring
- ❑ B base of the penis
- ❑ C thigh
- ❑ D superficial inguinal pouch
- ❑ E superficial inguinal ring

5.43 The following are true of testicular torsion:

- ❑ A peak age of incidence is ten years
- ❑ B it is more common in lower testes
- ❑ C it may be periodic
- ❑ D it may mimic epididymitis
- ❑ E it is associated with groin herniae

5.44 With regard to the prostate gland

- ❑ A benign prostatic hypertrophy occurs in the central zone
- ❑ B the peripheral zone is where malignancy mainly occurs
- ❑ C prostatitis affects the periurethral zone
- ❑ D in benign prostatic hypertrophy nodular hyperplasia occurs
- ❑ E the peripheral zone atrophies with age

5.45 The following are complications of TURP:

- ❑ A hypernatraemia
- ❑ B hypothermia
- ❑ C secondary haemorrhage
- ❑ D incontinence
- ❑ E increased risk of stroke

5.46 The following are presenting symptoms of prostatic cancer:

- ❑ A lower back pain
- ❑ B renal failure
- ❑ C haematospermia
- ❑ D diarrhoea
- ❑ E loin pain

5.47 Seminoma of the testis

- ❑ A is the most common testicular tumour
- ❑ B has a peak incidence between 20–30 years
- ❑ C spreads early via the bloodstream
- ❑ D is very sensitive to radiotherapy
- ❑ E has an overall cure rate of 90%

5.48 Teratoma of the testis

- ❑ A is associated with a hydrocele in 10% cases
- ❑ B has a later peak incidence than seminoma
- ❑ C spreads late via the bloodstream
- ❑ D recurrence may be monitored by α-fetoprotein and β-hCG
- ❑ E may present with a history of trauma

5.49 Renal calculi

- ❑ A usually present in the 40s
- ❑ B are usually due to hyperparathyroidism
- ❑ C may be caused by enterobacteria
- ❑ D in the renal pelvis may be treated with ESWL
- ❑ E produce microscopic haematuria in 50% cases

5.50 Extracorporeal shock wave lithotripsy (ESWL)

- ❑ A is the treatment for large staghorn calculi
- ❑ B should not be used for uric acid stones
- ❑ C may cause long-term renal damage
- ❑ D is complicated by sepsis in 10% cases
- ❑ E is used to treat stones in the upper 1/3 of the ureter
- ❑ F can be used in an obstructed kidney

5.51 Prostatic cancer

- ❑ A aminoglutethamide
- ❑ B cyproterone acetate
- ❑ C goserelin
- ❑ D stilboestrol
- ❑ E tamoxifen

Match the following with the above in the treatment of prostatic cancer.

1. anti-androgen
2. oestrogen
3. use in breast cancer
4. GnRH analogue
5. use with prednisolone

ANSWERS – SYSTEM MODULE A: LOCOMOTOR

1.1 Late complications of fractures **Answers: BCDE**

Infection is an early complication of fractures especially when open. Ideally, open fractures should be fixed within 4–6 hours of injury. Volkmann's ischaemic contracture occurs following arterial injury or compartment syndrome leading to claw hand or toes. Extensor pollicis longus rupture occurs late (6–12 weeks) after fracture of the lower radius and long head of biceps after humeral neck fracture. Myositis ossificans is heterotopic ossification in muscles especially after dislocation of the elbow or blow to brachialis, deltoid or quadriceps. Treatment includes rest then gentle active movements. Occasionally excision of the bony mass is required.

1.2 Fracture non-union **Answers: ABDE**

Non-union occurs as a result of unrecognised delayed union, wide separation of the fracture surfaces and soft tissue interposition. Painless movement at the fracture site is diagnostic of non-union as distinct from delayed union. Two types of non-union are described: hypertrophic (bulbous bone ends) and atrophic (no calcification at bone ends). Non-union is occasionally symptomless needing no treatment. Functional bracing may induce union and electrical stimulation may promote osteogenesis. Bone grafts are required for atrophic non-union.

1.3 Acute osteomyelitis **Answers: ACDE**

The features of acute osteomyelitis are pain, fever, inflammation, acute tenderness and normal X-rays if taken during the first ten days. After about ten days the area of infection appears mottled and a periosteal reaction begins. It can be very difficult to diagnose until relatively late in its course.

1.4 Rheumatoid arthritis **Answers: BDE**

Heberden's nodes occur in osteoarthritis and are tender distal interphalangeal joints. In rheumatoid arthritis there is usually symmetrical polyarthritis with early morning stiffness and raised ESR. The pathology follows a sequence of synovitis, joint destruction and deformity.

1.5 Rheumatoid arthritis **Answers: ACE**

Rheumatoid nodules are small granulomas found especially over bony prominences. Lymphadenopathy may affect any lymph node groups and the general reticuloendothelial system is activated leading to splenomegaly. Rheumatoid vasculitis can affect any organ but not infrequently causes renal failure.

1.6 Complications of rheumatoid arthritis **Answers: ABC**

Rheumatoid arthritis is a systemic disease and so can cause complications from vasculitis in any organ. Local complications include muscle weakness and joint contractures, joint ruptures, infection, amyloidosis and occasionally cord compression due to cervical instability (all patients with rheumatoid arthritis must have cervical spine views before a GA).

1.7 Delayed union of fractures **Answers: BCE**

Causes of delayed union include an inadequate blood supply, infection, incorrect immobilisation and intact fellow bone (such as the fibula in a tibial fracture). The fracture site is usually tender and the fracture remains visible with very little callus formation, periosteal reaction or sclerosis at the bone ends. Continued treatment is required and functional bracing is an excellent method of promoting bony union. If union is delayed for more than six months with no callus formation, then the fracture should undergo internal fixation and bone grafting.

1.8 Recurrent dislocation of patella **Answers: AC**

Predisposing factors to recurrent dislocation include generalised ligamentous laxity, underdevelopment of lateral femoral condyle and flattening of the intercondylar groove, maldevelopment of patella, valgus deformity and primary muscle defect. It is more common in girls and is often bilateral. Classically, patients whose patellae are moved laterally show great concern that it will dislocate – a positive 'apprehension test'.

1.9 Anterior knee pain **Answers: BCF**

Anterior knee pain is common amongst adolescents and adults and is often associated with softening and fibrillation of the articular surface of patella (chondromalacia patellae). It is probably due to mechanical overload of the patellofemoral joint.

1.10 Development of melanoma **Answers: ABE**

Clinical features are:

- changes in size, shape/outline (i.e. irregular)
- elevation (thicker, more palpable, nodules)
- colour (increasing pigmentation, irregular pigmentation and depigmentation)
- surrounding tissues, pigmented halo and satellite lesions
- development of symptoms, such as, itching, awareness, serous discharge and bleeding.

1.11 Good prognosis in malignant melanoma **Answer: B**

Male sex, increased tumour thickness, the presence of ulceration, older age and mucosal involvement are poor prognostic indicators. The prognosis also depends upon the lymph node involvement and growth pattern. The five-year survival rate is 90% for stage 1, 50% for stage II, 30% for stage III and < 1% for stage IV disease.

1.12 Acute septic arthritis of the knee **Answers: BCE**

Acute septic arthritis of the knee is not uncommon. The usual organism is *Staphylococcus aureus.* The joint is swollen, painful and inflamed. There is an elevated WBC and ESR. Pus may be aspirated. Systemic antibiotic should be started and irrigation of joint carried out. Should infection persist then osteoarthritis may result years later. Locking is associated with meniscal tears.

1.13 Ankylosing spondylitis **Answers: CD**

Ankylosing spondylitis is associated with HLA B27 (rheumatoid arthritis is HLA DR). It is more common in white males and may be associated with Reiter's disease and ulcerative colitis to give genito-urinary or gastrointestinal symptoms. Tests for rheumatoid factor (anti Ig-G) are negative.

1.14 X-ray features of osteoarthritis **Answers: AB**

There are four cardinal signs on an X-ray of osteoarthritis: asymmetrical joint space narrowing, sclerosis of subchondral bone, osteophytes and bone cysts.

1.15 Bone formation **Answers: BCE**

The immature state of bone is the woven one, this is then replaced by mature lamellar bone. The fibres in the latter are parallel to each other. Lamellar bone may be subdivided into cortical bone (e.g. the strong bone in the shaft of the femur) and the honeycomb inner bone or cancellous bone. This supports the marrow in the vertebrae and ends of the long bones.

1.16 Meniscal tears **Answers: ACE**

The meniscus is split along its length by force grinding it between the femur and tibia. The medial meniscus is affected much more frequently because its attachments to the capsule make it less mobile. A twisting injury to the semi-flexed knee is the typical form of injury. Most of the meniscus is avascular and spontaneous repair does not occur unless the tear is in the outer one-third that is vascularised from the capsule.

1.17 Paget's disease of the bone **Answers: BCDF**

Paget's disease of bone is characterised by enlargement and thickening of the bone but the internal architecture is abnormal and the bone is unusually brittle. It affects men and women equally especially from the age of 50 years. The most commonly affected sites are the pelvis and tibia. Complications include nerve compression, fractures, osteoarthritis, osteosarcoma, high output cardiac failure and hypercalcaemia.

1.18 Fall in serum calcium levels **Answers: BC**

Reduced serum calcium causes an increase in parathyroid hormone release. This in turn causes increased renal reabsorption of calcium and increased vitamin D production. Vitamin D then causes an increase in the intestinal absorption of calcium. Osteoclasts are also activated to increase bone resorption.

1.19 Calcium homeostasis **Answers: DE**

Calcitonin acts to oppose parathyroid hormone (PTH), i.e. it causes increased renal excretion and reduces bone resorption. Vitamin D produced in the skin by sunlight and ingested in the diet is firstly 25 hyroxylated in the liver and then 1 hyroxylated in the kidney to form the active 1,25 dihydroxycholecalciferol. This last stage is under the control of PTH and phosphorus. Oestrogen increases calcium absorption and protects against the effects of PTH.

1.20 Causes of osteoporosis **Answers: ABE**
Causes include malnutrition and malabsorption, hyperparathyroidism, Cushing's disease, (and syndrome from steroid administration) thyrotoxicosis and alcohol and heparin. Osteoporosis may also be caused by multiple myeloma, leukaemia, generalised carcinomatosis, rheumatoid arthritis, ankylosing spondylitis, TB and chronic renal disease. The most common cause however is menopause, iatrogenic or idiopathic.

1.21 Investigations for bone disease **Answers: ABCD**
As for any other disorder, a history must be taken looking for a menopausal history and causes for secondary metabolic bone disorder. Serum levels of calcium PTH, urinary calcium and phosphate should be taken. An IVU may show renal calculi if the patient is hypercalcaemic (bones, abdominal groans, stones, and moans).

1.22 Congenital dislocation of the hip **Answers: CDE**
Congenital dislocation of the hip is a phase of a spectrum of hip abnormality. It occurs in 5–20/1000 live births. Girls:boys 7:1 with the left hip affected more than the right. 1 in 5 cases is bilateral. It tends to run in families with the breech position favouring dislocation. Ultrasound will show the shape of the cartilaginous socket and position of the femoral head. It may present in adults (30–50 years) with increasing discomfort whereby backache and pain occur with walking.

1.23 Tuberculosis of the knee **Answers: AC**
Bone or joints are affected in about 5% of patients with TB. There is a predilection for vertebral bodies and large synovial joints. Granulation tissue may extend across the joint and articular cartilage causing bone erosion and local osteoporosis. There is little or no periosteal reaction. Synovial fluid yields the diagnosis in only 10–20% cases. Synovial biopsy is more reliable.

1.24 Paget's disease **Answer: B**
Paget's disease causes enlargement and thickening of bone. It mainly affects the tibia, femur, skull, spine and pelvis. Both sexes are affected equally. It usually presents after the 50th year. The enlarged bones are brittle and cause kyphotic, bow legged deformities. Cranial nerves may be compressed due to skull enlargement (VII, VIII, V). Alkaline phosphatase level is raised and used as a marker for disease activity. Malignant change occurs in about 1%.

1.25 Club-foot **Answers: AD**

Boys are twice as likely to be affected than girls. The feet are held in equinovarus i.e. downwards and inwards. The condition may be associated with spina bifida. The initial treatment is that of splintage, where the deformity is 'over corrected'. Resistant cases will require surgery in the form of a tendon release and fixation. Many operations have been described for the correction of club-foot.

1.26 Acute osteomyelitis **Answers: BCDE**

Acute osteomyelitis is most often found in children. In adults it is associated with immunosuppression and diabetes. The organism is most commonly *Staphylococcus aureus.* Others include *Strep. pyogenes* and *Strep. pneumoniae.* In children < 4 years *Haemophilus influenzae* is common. Organisms settle in the metaphysis, most often at the proximal end of the femur. In adults the thoracolumbar spine is the most common site.

1.27 Post-operative osteomyelitis **Answers: AC**

Osteomyelitis may occur after any operation on bone especially implantation of a prosthesis. The organisms may come from the atmosphere, instruments, patient, surgeon or indirectly from a distant focus. It may present early (within three months) or later. The organisms are usually a mixture of pathogenic bacteria (*S. aureus,* Proteus, Pseudomonas). Predisposing factors include soft tissue damage, bone death, poor contact between implant and bone, loosening and corrosion of the implant. Elimination of any focus of infection, optimal operative sterility, prophylactic antibiotics, close fit and secure fixation of implant all reduce the risk of post-operative osteomyelitis.

1.28 Carpal tunnel syndrome **Answers: ABE**

This is caused by compression and ischaemia of the median nerve. Pain and paraesthesia characteristically occur at night. It is associated with rheumatoid arthritis, pregnancy, hypothyroidism and is more common around the menopause. It occurs eight times more commonly in females. Froment's test is for ulnar nerve function, a positive Tinel's sign may be seen in carpal tunnel syndrome.

1.29 Hallux valgus **Answers: BCE**

Hallux valgus is a common condition affecting predominantly women. It usually presents at 50–70 years but there is an inherited variety presenting in adolescence. The treatment is surgical. Many operations have been suggested usually involving an osteotomy to correct the deformity.

1.30 Gout **Answers: CE**

The most common site is the metatarsophalangeal joint. The urate level is not always raised. The diagnostic test is that of joint aspiration and microscopy of the fluid collected. This fluid shows needle-shaped crystals which are negatively birefringent (reaction to polarised light under optical microscope).

1.31 Complications of hip replacement **Answers:**

A	death	2.	< 1%
B	pulmonary embolus, no prophylaxis	5.	10–20%
C	urinary retention male	1.	5–10%
D	DVT, no prophylaxis	4.	30–70%
E	wound infection without prophylaxis	3.	1–5%

Prophylaxis has had a vast impact on the reduction of deep wound infections and thrombotic complications. The risk of deep wound infection has dropped from 1–5% to < 1% and the risk of a DVT from 60% to 15%. The risk of a PE on low molecular weight heparin is 1–5%.

1.32 Rheumatoid hand **Answers: AD**

Synovitis occurs first in the metacarpophalangeal (MCP) and PIP joints and flexor and extensor tendon sheaths. There is radial deviation of the wrist and ulnar deviation of the hand. Swan neck deformity refers to hyperextension of the PIP and flexion of the DIP joint and boutonnière deformity refers to flexion deformity of the PIP joint. Rupture of the EPL gives rise to a mallet thumb. Heberden's nodes are found in osteoarthritis and are thickening of the DIP joint.

1.33 Dupuytren's contracture **Answers: AE**

This is nodular hypertrophy and contracture of the superficial palmar fascia. It is also associated with plantar aponeurosis thickening and fibrosis of corpus cavernosum (Peyronie's disease). It is associated with alcoholic cirrhosis, diabetes mellitus, vibrating machinery and tuberculosis. Usually affects the ring finger first. The digital nerve is displaced but not invaded. Operation is indicated if the deformity is a nuisance or rapidly progressing. Fasciectomy or excision of thickened fascia is the usual operation. Amputation is occasionally needed if there is severe contracture that the patient finds disabling.

1.34 Humeral shaft fractures **Answers: BCD**

Injury to the radial nerve is common but recovery is usual. Fractures of the humerus heal readily and require neither perfect reduction nor immobilisation. The weight of the arm with an external cast is usually enough to pull the fragments into alignment. Spiral fractures unite in six weeks, other varieties in 10–12 weeks. Delayed union may occur in transverse fractures. Child abuse must be considered in humeral shaft fractures.

1.35 Frozen shoulder **Answers: BD**

Frozen shoulder or supraspinatus tendinitis is due to inflammation of the supraspinatus tendon. It classically has a painful arc of movement between 60–120° of abduction. Treatment involves, rest, ice, NSAIDs, and steroid and local anaesthetic injections on the antero-lateral acromial region.

1.36 Perthes' disease **Answers: CE**

This disease affects boys:girls 4:1. It presents between the ages of 4–8 years when the child has a painful limp. The condition is due to avascular necrosis of the femoral head. The presentation peak coincides with change from femoral shaft vessels to ligamentum teres vessels to supply the head. It is more common in caucasian boys of social class V.

1.37 Supracondylar fracture **Answers: BDE**

Supracondylar fractures are usually seen in children. There is usually posterior displacement of the fragment due to a fall on an outstretched hand. The jagged end of the proximal fragment pokes into the tissues anteriorly injuring the brachial artery or median nerve. Compartment syndrome may ensue. The median nerve injury is usually temporary and recovery can be expected in 6–8 weeks. Malunion is common.

1.38 Combined fracture of radius and ulna **Answers: BE**

These types of injuries are common in RTA. In children the fracture is often incomplete and only angulated. Closed reduction is usually successful in children. In adults, unless the fragments are in close apposition, reduction is difficult and redisplacement in the cast is almost invariable hence open reduction and internal fixation is favoured by most surgeons. Nerve injury due to the fracture is rare. There is good collateral circulation thus injury to radial or ulnar artery seldom presents any problem.

1.39 Slipped femoral epiphysis **Answers: AC**

This condition occurs at the age of 12–16 years with a male preponderance. It is more common on the left than the right. The slip leads to an externally rotated leg and coxa vara.

1.40 Dislocation of hip **Answers: ACD**

1.41 Colles' fracture **Answers: ABDE**

A Colles' fracture is a transverse fracture of the radius just above the wrist with dorsal displacement of the distal fragment. Nerve injury is rare. Reflex sympathetic dystrophy is quite common. Malunion and stiffness of the shoulder are common complications.

1.42 Internal fixation **Answers: ABCE**

Internal fixation is often the most desirable form of treatment. The main indications are fractures that are unstable, unite slowly, pathological fractures or where there may be nursing difficulties. Fixation of multiple fractures reduces the risk of general complications and late multiple organ failure. If the bones have been fixed rigidly with the ends apart, the fracture may fail to unite. Iatrogenic infection is now the most common cause of chronic osteitis.

1.43 Bone grafts **Answers: ABE**

Bone grafts are either autogenous or homografts. Cancellous bone grafts can provide linkage by filling cavities or replacing crushed bone. Cortical bone can provide splintage e.g. in treating non-union or arthrodesing a joint. Fresh allografts induce an inflammatory response in the individual and may lead to rejection. Antigenicity may be reduced by freezing or freeze drying or by ionising radiation. Donors must be cleared of malignancy, syphilis, hepatitis and HIV.

1.44 Osteoid osteoma **Answer: C**

These benign tumours have no malignant potential. They are very painful, however the pain responds very well to salicylates. The treatment is surgical, however the localisation of these small lesions can be difficult. They show up very well on a bone scan.

1.45 Bone tumours **Answer: C**

Brown tumours of bone are associated with hyperparathyroidism. Aneurysmal bone cysts occur at the metaphysis and are eccentric and expand. Breast metastases are usually porotic, however, in keeping with prostatic secondary disease they may be sclerotic. Prostatic secondaries may also be porotic.

ANSWERS – SYSTEM MODULE B: VASCULAR

2.1 Calf claudication **Answers: CDE**

Claudication is worse in the cold and walking uphill (spinal claudication is improved by walking uphill). The claudication classically resolves on rest and may initially be associated with muscle spasm. The symptoms may present without significant arterial disease in the case of popliteal entrapment.

2.2 Acute arterial occlusion **Answers: BDE**

If acute occlusion occurs in the absence of chronic disease then there are very few collaterals formed. This means that the tissue distal to the occlusion is rendered ischaemic and so cold, painful, paraesthetic, pale and pulseless. This will then lead to infarction if the perfusion is not returned to the organ. Bier spots are the white blotches that appear amongst the blue/purple discoloration.

2.3 Acute ischaemia **Answers: CE**

Nerve conduction disappears after about 30 minutes of complete ischaemia, permanent muscle injury then follows after a few hours if circulation is not restored. In established ischaemia there is a risk of reperfusion injury where toxins are liberated into the blood and can cause cardiac arrest or renal failure.

2.4 Venous ulceration **Answers: AD**

Klippel-Trenauney syndrome is characterised by a cutaneous naevus, varicose veins, and bone and soft tissue hypertrophy affecting one or more limbs. There are no pathological arteriovenous fistulae. Venous ulceration should be managed by conservative means first because the majority (80%) heal within one year with paste bandages and elastic compression. Stripping of the superficial veins is contraindicated if the deep system is thrombosed. Female:male ratio of 2:1. Squamous cell carcinoma (Marjolin's ulcer) occurs in long standing non-healing ulcers.

2.5 Ischaemic rest pain **Answers: AE**

Rest pain classically occurs at night time when it is proposed the cardiac output falls and so worsens ischaemia. The patient is woken with a cold painful foot/toes and puts them out of the bed or walks around to relieve the pain. The limb will show muscle wasting and the skin will be hairless and thinned due to chronic vascular insufficiency.

2.6 Mesenteric ischaemia **Answers: BCD**

Mesenteric ischaemia is a very difficult diagnosis and usually follows the exclusion of many other diagnoses. Classically a patient will present with weight loss, bloody diarrhoea and pain after eating. This pain is cramping in nature. The patient may also have features of other vascular disease. They may have an epigastric bruit.

2.7 The spleen **Answers: AE**

Splenomegaly may occur as part of Felty's syndrome (rheumatoid arthritis, granulocytopenia and splenomegaly) where antibodies against granulocytes lead to recurrent infections in non-healing leg ulcers. In ITP anti-platelet antibodies (IgG) lead to purpura. Hepatic failure if caused by cirrhosis, splenic or portal vein thrombosis may be associated with splenomegaly. Hypersplenism is usually defined as the combination of splenomegaly, cytopenia, marrow hyperplasia and subsequent improvement after splenectomy. Patients with sickle cell disease have chronic splenic infarction leading to a small non-functioning spleen. Both leukaemia and lymphoma may be associated with splenomegaly.

2.8 Primary lymphoedema of the legs **Answers: CD**

In primary lymphoedema, the cause is intrinsic to lymphatic development, whereas in secondary lymphoedema there is a separate causative process such as trauma, malignant disease, irradiation, infection or inflammation. Anatomically, there are no lymphatic vessels in the epidermis, even in normal subjects. Malignant infiltration of inguinal lymph nodes/lymphatics is a common cause of secondary lymphoedema of the legs. The skin of patients with primary lymphoedema is often hyperkeratotic and thick so ulceration is not common. However, vesicles and fistulas producing pure lymph may form and be successfully treated by conservative measures. Operative treatment of such minor lymph leaks is usually reserved for the rarer resistant cases. In the past, diuretics have been extensively used to treat lymphoedema, but they are probably of little use because the increased limb volume is composed more of protein and fibrotic tissue than of water.

2.9 Vascular disease **Answers: ABC**

It is important to assess for anaemia or hyperviscosity. A raised ESR may indicate a vasculitic cause. Although syphilis is rare today, it can catch out the unwary. (VDRL - Venereal Disease Research Laboratory.)

2.10 Arterial disease **Answers: BCE**

Plethysmography is largely a research tool. Greyscale ultrasound has found its place in the assessment of arterial disease and combined with Doppler in duplex scanning is a very useful tool. Thallium scanning may be used to assess cardiac disease as can electrocardiography and exercise testing. CT scans may be used to assess aneurysms.

2.11 Carotid artery stenosis **Answer: B**

Carotid artery stenosis may cause embolisation or thrombotic occlusion leading to transient ischaemic attack, ischaemic stroke or retinal infarct. A patient with asymptomatic carotid stenosis with a reduction in luminal diameter of 50% has a risk of 1–2% per year of developing a stroke. Bruits are an unreliable guide to presence or severity of carotid stenosis – 37% accuracy for diagnosis of moderate/severe stenosis. Duplex ultrasound may fail to distinguish severe stenosis from occlusion. Mild to moderate symptomatic carotid stenosis derives no benefit of stroke prevention from endarterectomy.

2.12 Surgical treatments for lymphoedema **Answers: ABE**

Operations for lymphoedema can be classified into reducing or bypass operations. In reducing operations, the lymphodematous subcutaneous tissue and skin are excised. In bypass operations, the sites of localised lymphatic obstruction are bypassed. Examples of reducing operations include Charles' and Homan's operations. Kinmonth's mesenteric bridge operation is an example of bypass procedures.

2.13 Rest pain but no gangrene **Answers: BCDE**

The Doppler index is the leg pressure over the arm pressure in mmHg taken using a Doppler ultrasound probe to ascultate the pulse and a sphygmomanometer cuff to occlude inflow. Normal is 1.0 to 1.2, claudication starts at about 0.8, rest pain at 0.4 and gangrene when it falls further. The Doppler signal is also of value in that the normal waveform is triphasic, as disease progresses it becomes biphasic and then monophasic.

2.14 Translumbar aortography — Answers: AB

Translumbar aortography has largely been superseded by the retrograde Seldinger technique. The main complications are dissection, embolism, false aneurysm formation, thrombosis and haemorrhage. It is for this reason that it is not without risk to the patient. With modern less ionic contrast media, reactions are rare.

2.15 Arteriovenous fistulae — Answers: AB

Branham's test is where occlusion of the feeding vessel to a large arteriovenous fistula causes bradycardia due to the reversal of the large left to right shunt. These lesions deteriorate during puberty and pregnancy. In Klippel-Trenauney syndrome there are mesodermal deformities with naevae and lymphatic abnormality, a persistent lateral vein of the thigh gives rise to gross varicose veins.

2.16 Carotid endarterectomy — Answers: BCDE

5% of patients who undergo endarterectomy for symptomatic carotid stenosis have a stroke or die within 30 days of the operation. Patients are more likely to suffer from peri-operative stroke/death if they are female, > 75 years, have peripheral vascular disease, history of cerebral TIA, occlusion of contralateral internal carotid artery or stenosis of the ipsilateral external carotid artery. There is a 3% risk of peri-operative myocardial infarction.

2.17 Carotid endarterectomy — Answers: A

Only patients with severe carotid (> 70%) stenosis who have recently become symptomatic have been demonstrated to derive worthwhile benefit from surgery. Most surgeons would consider a large completed stroke as a contraindication for surgery.

2.18 Peripheral vascular disease — Answers: ABCDF

All patients with peripheral vascular disease should have a FBC, urea and electrolytes, glucose (random blood). ESR may be elevated in collagen diseases, Buerger's disease and inflammatory aneurysms. Elevated serum cholesterol should be treated to prevent rapid progression of the disease. Echocardiography is useful to confirm cardiac valvular disease, LV function and possible thrombus in the atrium or LV. Plethysmography is essentially a research tool.

2.19 Strawberry patch **Answers: CD**

The congenital cavernous haemangioma (strawberry patch) will resolve spontaneously in about 60% of cases. These lesions may ulcerate and bleed and calcify, if large then they can cause a consumptive coagulopathy. They usually need several treatments with cryotherapy.

2.20 Cervical rib **Answers: BDE**

Cervical rib is present in about 0.5% of the population where 60% are symptomatic. The most common presentation is that of neurological symptoms of paraesthesia in the T1 nerve distribution. Emboli or spasm may cause digital gangrene.

2.21 Traumatic bleeding **Answers: BD**

Bleeding following trauma to a major vessel is best controlled by direct pressure. The use of ligation should be avoided unless under direct vision in the operating theatre. Angiography is unhelpful in large haemorrhage but may be helpful if performed on table to assess distal flow and run off. Vein patching is not always necessary.

2.22 Arteriovenous fistulae **Answers: ABDE**

AV fistulae may be a rare cause of bacterial endocarditis. If large enough they can cause significant venous hypertension and so lipodermatosclerosis and ulceration.

2.23 Carotid endarterectomy **Answers: BC**

The untreated stroke rate for all transient ischaemic attacks is about 5% at one year. There is good evidence for treating symptomatic severe stenoses > 70%. Trials are being conducted regarding asymptomatic greater stenoses and the symptomatic lower stenotic groups. The stroke rate and mortality of surgery should be below 2% and ideally less than 1%.

2.24 Monitoring patient during endarterectomy **Answers: BD**

Measuring the distal stump pressure is used to see how adequate the collateral circulation is. The operation can also be performed under local anaesthetic and so the patient is easily monitored with regard to ischaemic events. Shunting is not a form of monitoring.

2.25 Acute lower limb ischaemia **Answers: ABD**

Diabetic patients may have peripheral sensorineuropathy and therefore experience less pain in the midst of ischaemia. Acute sensorimotor impairment is not irreversible but is an indication for urgent action. Colour changes do not themselves signify irreversible ischaemia provided that there is blanching on pressure. Fasciotomy is an operation that must not be delayed and is indicated if there is evidence of motor loss and induration in a group of muscles.

2.26 Atheroma **Answers: CD**

Atheroma is focal intimal damage consisting of fibrous tissue and lipid with smooth muscle proliferation. It mainly affects the medium and large arteries. A fatty streak leads to a fibrolipid plaque. This is then infiltrated with foamy macrophages which damage the endothelium further. Platelet derived growth factor is released and stimulates the smooth muscle proliferation. Increased LDL cholesterol with a reduced HDL and diabetes together with intimal damage caused by hypertension, nicotine and adrenaline increase atheroma. Oestrogens protect (low rates of disease for pre-menopausal women).

2.27 Graft patency rates

A	reversed vein fem-pop graft	1.	70%
B	fem-pop dacron graft patency	4.	45%
C	aorto-fem patency	5.	90%
D	axillo-femoral patency	3.	60%
E	fem-fem cross-over patency	2.	80%

Patency rates at five years are related to the force and volume of inflow and the run off away from the graft. If run off is poor then even though the blood goes into the graft it may have nowhere to go and so stagnates and leads to graft occlusion and failure. Synthetic grafts below the inguinal ligament are vastly inferior to vein.

2.28 Amputations **Answers: CE**

90% of amputations are carried out for ischaemia. Especially in diabetic ischaemic feet the skin flaps should be left open to allow free drainage and no tension should be placed on the wound. Chopart described a transmetatarsal amputation and so is useless for an ischaemic heel. AKA should have a 30 cm stump and BKA 15 cm stump (approx). The Burgess BKA utilises a long posterior flap.

2.29 Common iliac artery **Answer: B**

The common iliac artery extends from the division of the abdominal aorta on the left side of the body of L4 to the sacroiliac joint where it divides into the external and internal iliac arteries. The sympathetic trunk is posterior to the common iliac artery but the ureter is anterior.

2.30 External iliac artery **Answers: BD**

The external iliac artery becomes the common femoral artery beyond the inguinal ligament. It is crossed by the gonadal vessels and the ductus deferens/round ligament. The external iliac artery has two large branches: inferior epigastric artery and the deep circumflex iliac artery.

2.31 Femoral sheath **Answers: BD**

This is 3–4 cm long formed by the fascia iliaca posteriorly and the fascia transversalis anteriorly. The sheath is divided into three compartments, the lateral contains the femoral artery, the middle the femoral vein and the medial compartment the femoral canal. The femoral nerve lies outside the femoral sheath.

2.32 Aneurysms **Answers: DE**

The elective mortality rates for abdominal aortic aneurysms should be less than 5%. For emergency the mortality rate rises to 50%. At present there is no proven benefit for replacing aortas below 5 cm in diameter. (A small aneurysm study is continuing at present).

2.33 Raynaud's phenomenon **Answers: ABDE**

Raynaud's syndrome usually affects young women (60–90%) and causes intermittent cold blue extremities, usually fingers. This may cause trophic finger changes and even gangrene. The disease may be primary or secondary. Secondary causes include connective tissue disorders (SLE, CREST, PAN, RA), arterial disease, blood disorders including cold agglutinins and polycythaemia. The condition may also be associated with the contraceptive pill and beta blockers.

2.34 Femoral artery **Answers: AD**

The femoral artery lies in the lateral compartment of the femoral sheath and passes behind sartorius into the adductor canal. The artery lies on the floor of the femoral triangle – iliopsoas, pectineus and adductor longus. The profunda femoris arises from the upper lateral aspect of the femoral artery. Through the profunda femoris artery there is an arterial supply to the buttock and anastomosis behind the knee.

2.35 Management of the diabetic foot **Answers: ACDE**

Control of the sepsis and diabetes is of paramount importance. The use of systemic antibiotics is required initially parenterally. Flexor tendons and fascia are common routes by which infection may spread. Drainage of collections should be carried out.

2.36 Acute arterial embolism **Answers: AE**

The effect of embolic occlusion of an artery depends upon the site, speed of onset, pre-existence of disease and potential for collateral supply. There is no evidence that thrombolysis with or without angioplasty is superior to open embolectomy. One or both groins should be exposed from which site saddle thrombus and distal emboli can be retrieved via Fogarty catheters (size 4 or 5 and 3, respectively). The arteriotomy should be closed with a monofilament polypropylene suture.

2.37 Glomus tumours **Answers: CD**

These are benign tumours. They are equally common in men and women and occur on the fingers in half the patients. They are almost invariably painful. Subungual tumours can be difficult to detect but may cause rarefaction of the distal phalanx on X-ray. The treatment is surgical excision.

2.38

A	Kaposi's sarcoma	4.	blue red macule with HIV
B	angiosarcoma	3.	rapid growing, bulky
C	chemodectoma	1.	carotid artery
D	glomus jugulare tumour	5.	buzzing in head
E	leiomyomas	2.	more common in veins than arteries

2.39 Complications of varicose veins **Answers: ABCE**
Varicose veins are more common after deep vein thrombosis. They may cause lipodermatosclerosis, which if left may then ulcerate, the medial maleolar region being the most common site for this. There should be no paraesthesia, but they can spontaneously rupture causing brisk bleeding.

2.40 Arterial stenosis **Answer: C**
Constriction of an artery increases the velocity of the blood through the constriction, producing turbulence beyond the constriction. Flow rate decreases when stenosis exceeds 70%. Resistance is proportional to the radius to the 4th power (r^4).

2.41 The popliteal fossa **Answers: CDE**
The medial side of the popliteal fossa is formed from the semitendinosus and semimembranosus muscles. The biceps femoris forms the lateral side passing to the head of the fibula. The common peroneal nerve is the second main division of the sciatic and enters the popliteal fossa at its apex and passes downwards and laterally deep to biceps femoris and superficial to the lateral head of gastrocnemius. The tibial nerve gives off sensory branches – sural nerve and branches to the knee joint.

2.42 Major lower limb amputation **Answers: ABD**
There is an increased incidence of DVT in patients requiring amputations from all causes. Antibiotics covering staphylococci and *Clostridium perfringens* should be administered. If there is concern over anaerobes then metronidazole should be added. Below knee amputation can be performed either by a skew flap technique (equal anteromedial and posterolateral flaps) or a long posterior flap (Burgess). 48 hours of pre-op analgesia in the form of an epidural has been shown to reduce phantom limb pain.

2.43 Abdominal aortic aneurysm (AAA) **Answers: BCE**
98% of abdominal aortic aneurysm are infra-renal. AAA are most common in men aged over 60 years who have hypertension and who smoke. The imaging methods of choice are ultrasound and CT. Arteriography is used to assess the renal arteries. Small aneurysm trials are presently underway to assess whether AAA < 4 cm should be repaired.

2.44 Popliteal artery aneurysm **Answers: CDE**

Popliteal artery aneurysm is the second most common site for artery aneurysm formation. It usually presents with ischaemia from embolisation of thrombus or thrombosis of the aneurysm. Diagnosis is confirmed by arteriography, ultrasound or CT. Fibrinolysis is used occasionally to lyse the thrombus before the aneurysm is repaired.

2.45 Varicose veins **Answers: ACD**

Varicose veins may be truly congenital with an inherited condition of absent valves. Many patients have a familial history, however, after a deep vein thrombosis one must assess the deep system to establish that this is present and competent. Both duplex and venography are useful in assessing disease and eliciting the exact site of incompetence prior to surgery.

2.46 Venous ulcers **Answers: BCE**

Venous ulcers have a sloping edge, a raised edge may indicate malignancy of a squamous or basal cell carcinoma. Any ulcer may become malignant and so biopsies must be taken from longstanding ulceration (Marjolin's ulcer). A positive WR (Wasserman reaction) may indicate that the ulcer is due to syphilis.

2.47 Deep vein thrombosis (DVT) **Answers: BCD**

Smoking appears to reduce the incidence of DVT. Venography and ultrasound are the main diagnostic tools available (with a good history and clinical examination!). Research tools include radiolabelled fibrinogen studies.

2.48 Recurrent TIA **Answers: ABE**

Atherosclerosis is the most common pathology of carotid artery disease. Other rare causes of transient neurological events include arteritis, trauma and aneurysmal disease. A heterogeneous plaque, critical or severe stenosis should prompt intravenous DSA. Selective catheterisation should be avoided if possible as this can occasionally dislodge plaque-derived emboli.

2.49 External carotid artery **Answers: ABF**

The terminal division of the external carotid artery, superficial temporal and maxillary arteries within the parotid gland. The occipital and posterior auricular artery branches pass along the lower and upper borders of posterior belly of digastric. Through the pharyngeal artery, the external carotid artery supplies the meninges.

2.50 Femoral artery aneurysm **Answers: BCD**

Femoral artery aneurysm usually presents with a pulsatile mass. Any groin surgery involving exposure of the femoral artery may be complicated by lymph fistula.

2.51 Factors increasing risk of DVT **Answers: ABD**

Inherited deficiencies of natural inhibitors of coagulation including anti-thrombin III, protein C, protein S, activated protein C (Leiden factor) are associated with DVT. Sickle cell is also associated with arterial thrombosis, but not DVT.

ANSWERS – SYSTEM MODULE C: HEAD, NECK, ENDOCRINE AND PAEDIATRIC

3.1 Tumours of the thyroid region — Answers: ACD

Medullary thyroid tumours release calcitonin and so this forms a convenient way to monitor patient progress. The radionucleotide scans, of which the technetium based sestaMIBI scan is one, are used in both localising and monitoring parathyroid tumours. MRI, CT and thallium/technetium subtraction scans are also used.

3.2 Cleft lip — Answers: ABD

Cleft lip is on the increase with 1/750 live births being affected. The condition is more common in male births. The subsequent risk that other children will be affected, given that the first born has a cleft lip, is 5% rising to 9% with two affected siblings.

3.3 Cleft palate — Answers: ABD

Cleft palate is associated with hearing loss due to the increased risk of middle ear infections. Speech recovers after repair in about 75% providing the repair is between the ages of six months and one year, to allow the best chance of speech developing normally.

3.4 Assessment of thyroid enlargement — Answers: AE

Ultrasonography is operator dependent but can identify nodules as small as 0.3 mm in diameter. It can differentiate cystic from solid lesions, but not benign from malignant disease. Isotope scanning (^{123}I or ^{99m}Tc) has a role in investigating solitary autonomous nodule or toxic multinodular goitre, identifying metastatic thyroid tumour and localisation of ectopic thyroid tissue. FNAC can accurately diagnose a colloid nodule, thyroiditis, papillary carcinoma, lymphoma and anaplastic carcinoma.

3.5 Dissection of neck **Answer: B**

Primary hyperparathyroidism (PHPT) is relatively common in the UK, being four times more common in women than in men. There is a high concentration of parathyroid hormone, inappropriate to the level of ionised calcium in the plasma. The usual cause is a parathyroid adenoma. A normal parathyroid gland may be mistaken for fat because of its yellowish brown colour. The superior parathyroid glands are usually found behind the middle third of the thyroid lobes, in close proximity to the recurrent laryngeal nerve and above the inferior thyroid artery. The inferior parathyroid glands are more variable in position but are most often located on the posterolateral surface of the inferior pole of the thyroid gland, inferior to the inferior thyroid artery. In PHPT all four glands may be enlarged, but it is most usual for there to be a single adenoma with the other glands appearing normal. Ectopic calcification in the tissues of the neck is not usually a feature of PHPT.

3.6 Tumours of the hypothalamus **Answers: ABCDE**

Hypothalamic tumours not only produce neuroendocrine problems but also symptoms of increased intracranial pressure, epilepsy, chiasmal compression or hydrocephalus. Such lesions also affect appetite, temperature and mood and interfere with the drainage of CSF.

3.7 Cranial tumours **Answers: BCDE**

Headache associated with brain tumours is frequently noticeable in the early morning and is often exacerbated by movement or coughing. Changes in alertness or mood may be reported by patient's relatives or friends. Partial III and IV nerve palsies occur with incipient brain herniation at the tentorial notch – patients complain of diplopia on lateral gaze. Rarely the first noticeable effect of tumour will be the sudden brain herniation with coning at the tentorium or foramen magnum resulting in an apnoeic attack – urgent treatment and investigations are indicated.

3.8 Carcinoma of the parotid gland **Answers: ABC**

The risk factors for carcinoma of the parotid gland include pleomorphic adenoma, breast cancer and previous radiotherapy. The histological grade is more predictive of prognosis and behaviour than the histological type. The diagnosis is usually confirmed by core biopsy (or FNAC). The mainstay of the treatment is surgical excision. Radiotherapy is indicated for high grade lesions. The 10-year survival rate is 90% for low grade tumours and 25% for high grade ones.

3.9 *Herpes simplex*

A	*Herpes simplex*	3.	cold sore
B	candidiasis	5.	thrush
C	beta haemolytic streptococcus	4.	Ludwig's angina
D	fusospirochaetal infection	1.	Vincent's angina
E	*Treponema pallidum*	2.	gumma

3.10 Squamous cell carcinoma **Answers: ACDE**

Cigarette smoking or alcohol intake may have a synergistic relationship in the development of oral cancer, although there is little evidence for this. Pipe smoking may be connected. Syphilis is no longer considered to be one of the associated conditions with oral neoplasia. The condition is more common in Sri Lanka and India.

3.11 Papillary carcinoma of the thyroid **Answers: ADF**

The most common presentation of papillary carcinoma is a thyroid nodule frequently associated with enlarged cervical lymph nodes. 85% of irradiation-induced tumours are papillary. Children and young adults are the population at greatest risk. Papillary carcinoma spreads to the paratracheal and cervical lymph nodes. It is frequently multifocal (30–87%) and rarely encapsulated. Blood borne spread is usually a late feature.

3.12 Carcinoma of the lip **Answers: BDE**

The incidence of lip cancer is higher among caucasians, smokers and outdoor workers. SCC is the most common histological type. Basal cell carcinoma is occasionally seen. 92% of lesions occur in the lower lip, 5% in the upper lip and 3% at the angle of the mouth. Surgery and radiotherapy are equally effective.

3.13 Medullary carcinoma of the thyroid **Answers: CDEF**

Medullary carcinoma of the thyroid may present with a stony hard lump in the upper half of the gland with or without cervical lymph node metastases. It is sporadic in 80% of cases and familial in 20%. It has an association with MEN type IIA and IIB. The parafollicular cells produce calcitonin protein which is deposited as amyloid.

3.14 Thyroid cancer **Answers: BCE**

Chemotherapy is not effective. Dissection of the involved lymph nodes only (berry picking) is required.

3.15 Thyroglossal tract **Answers: BCD**

The thyroglossal tract is the remnant of the path the thyroid takes as it descends. It starts at the foramen caecum of the tongue where the filiform and valate papillae meet. It then traverses the hyoid bone to be continuous with the pyramidal lobe of the thyroid gland.

3.16 Thyroglossal cyst **Answers: ABC**

Classically thyroglossal cysts are in the midline and can arise from any part of the track. They are lined by stratified squamous epithelium or ciliated pseudostratified epithelium. Both pouches and cystic hygromata are away from the midline and are generally soft in texture.

3.17 Simple goitre **Answers: ABC**

Simple goitre is caused by either a deficiency of iodine or a relative increase in demand, or a failure of the enzyme system. Antithyroid drugs and radiation may also cause it. The most frequent cause is a physiological one due to increased demand during pregnancy or puberty. *E. coli* when it infects drinking water may produce thiopyramine nucleotide, a strongly goitrogenic substance.

3.18 Thyrotoxicosis **Answers: BD**

Graves' disease accounts for about 90% of thyrotoxicosis. This is more common in women (10:1) and is caused by thyroid stimulating immunoglobulins. Thyrotoxicosis is a multi-system disease affecting all organs.

- **General** – weight loss, increased appetite, fever, sweating, heat intolerance.
- **CVS** – palpitations, angina, failure, atrial fibrillation
- **Neurological** – tremor, psychosis, proximal myopathy, myasthenia, choreoathetosis
- **GIT** – vomiting, diarrhoea, steatorrhoea
- **Skin** – hyperpigmentation, acropachy, spider naevi, palmar erythema, pretibial myxoedema
- **Bones** – osteoporosis, eye changes, reproductive, oligomenorrhoea, gynaecomastia.

3.19 Tumours related to smoking **Answers: ACE**

Bladder, cervical and laryngeal cancer are all smoking related. No such association exists for the leukaemias and lymphomas.

3.20 Investigation of a thyroid lump **Answers: AE**

The routine investigation includes history, examination, thyroid ultrasound, fine needle aspiration cytology as well as thyroid function tests and an autoantibody screen.

3.21 Lump in right thyroid lobe **Answers: BD**

This woman should have a full clinical examination followed by an ultrasound scan. She should also be shown to be chemically euthyroid. The scan will show if the lump is solid or cystic, or part of a multinodular picture. If the lump is solid then fine needle aspiration should be carried out. If this is done prior to the scan then it may change the picture and so should be deferred.

3.22 Multi-nodular colloid goitre (MNCG) Answers: ADE

The usual presentation of a MNCG is that of an unsightly unwanted cosmetic appearance. Patients are usually euthyroid although some may be hyperthyroid. There may be discomfort or even features of tracheal or oesophageal compression. All patients should have thyroid function checked and an ultrasound scan. Technetiun scanning will help show any retrosternal extension and show if there is a component of a hot or cold nodule. CT scanning may be helpful only if malignancy is suspected and so the capsule can be examined to look for extracapsular extension. CT may also help if a complex retrosternal goitre is noted.

3.23 Tumour of the thyroid gland Answers: CE

The tumours of the thyroid may be classified as benign or malignant and primary or secondary. The benign tumours include follicular adenoma, and teratoma. The malignant tumours are 1) differentiated tumours: medullary, follicular, papillary, mixed carcinomas, 2) anaplastic, 3) lymphoma, 4) sarcoma, teratoma, squamous cell. The assessment of these lesions includes ultrasound scanning and FNAC. The diagnosis of a follicular carcinoma (and not adenoma) relies on extension of the cells beyond the capsule and so cannot be made on FNAC. Medullary carcinoma is part of the MEN II syndrome.

3.24 Thyroid disease

A	hot nodule	3.	Plummer's syndrome
B	lymphoma	1.	radiotherapy and chemotherapy
C	follicular adenoma	4.	hemi-thyroidectomy only
D	anaplastic carcinoma	2.	resection and radiotherapy
E	follicular carcinoma	5.	total thyroidectomy and radio iodine

The condition of a solitary hot functioning nodule is Plummer's syndrome and accounts for 5% of all cases of thyrotoxicosis. Follicular adenomas only need resection. However if the histology shows carcinoma then the patient should have a completion thyroidectomy and radio iodine treatment.

3.25 Inguinal hernia **Answers: BEF**

10% of inguinal hernia in children present with irreducible hernias and the risk of this is highest in the first three months of life. Prompt elective surgery is essential. Simple herniotomy will suffice as the inguinal canal develops its obliquity at the age of 11–12 years. Delivering the testicle into the wound leads to much higher complications such as ischaemia.

3.26 Laryngeal nerve **Answer: C**

The recurrent laryngeal nerves are sensory to the subglottic region and supply all the intrinsic muscles except cricothyroid.

3.27 Following a thyroidectomy **Answers: CE**

The use of drains in thyroidectomy is useful however they can occlude and they do not take the place of full haemostasis pre-closure. Drains do not always prevent clot formation causing respiratory distress, they may however give a guide to the amount of bleeding. In complete RLN section the cords assume the cadaveric position of slight abduction, in partial division they are fully adducted and so more obstructive. Hypocalcaemia may occur post surgery due to calcitonin release or complete removal of all parathyroid tissue.

3.28

A	propylthiouracil	4.	safe in breast feeding
B	^{131}I	1.	concentrated in toxic nodules
C	carbimazole	2.	agranulocytosis
D	dexamethasone	5.	thyroid crisis
E	thyroxine	3.	multinodular goitre

3.29 Respiratory distress following thyroidectomy **Answers: BCE**

Unilateral cord paralysis does not cause distress on its own, the patient may not notice the vocal effects unless they have a trained voice. Tracheomalacia is where the trachea is soft and so after the surgery may collapse. The treatment for this is intubation.

3.30 Excess parathyroid hormone **Answers: BC**

The biological effects of excessive PTH are decreased excretion of calcium by kidney associated with increased excretion of sodium, potassium and bicarbonate. There is increased absorption of calcium by direct action of the hormone on GI cells and indirectly through increased renal synthesis of 1,25 dihydrocholecalciferol. Increased resorption of bone leads to osteitis fibrosa cystica and subperiosteal phalangeal erosions.

3.31 Parathyroid glands **Answers: ADE**

The parathyroid glands originate from the 3rd and 4th branchial pouches with the lower glands coming from the 3rd pouch and the upper the 4th. The glands are symmetrical in about 80% of cases. The lower gland positioning is more variable with 30% located in the thymus gland and 3% being absent.

3.32

A	primary hyperparathyroidism	3.	adenoma
B	secondary hyperparathyroidism	4.	renal disease
C	tertiary hyperparathyroidism	2.	normal serum calcium
D	parathyroid hormone	1.	osteoclast
E	hypoparathyroidism	5.	thyroid surgery

Hyperparathyroidism in the primary situation is caused by an adenoma in 80% of cases, the rest are due to hyperplasia of the glands (19%) or a carcinoma (1%). Secondary disease is due to a chronic calcium deficiency usually as a result of chronic renal impairment. Tertiary disease is when the parathyroid glands become autonomous as a result of long term stimulation from secondary disease.

3.33 Hypercalcaemia **Answers: ADE**

There are many causes of raised serum calcium levels. The most common are multiple myeloma, skeletal metastatic tumour deposits and primary hyperparathyroidism. Other causes include thyrotoxicosis, Paget's disease of the bone, sarcoidosis, vitamin D intoxication, milk alkali syndrome, Addison's disease, thiazide diuretics, TB and familial.

3.34 Hyperparathyroidism **Answers: BCD**

Hyperparathyroidism presents with bone features of brown tumours, phalangeal tufting and pepper-potting of the skull. Due to the raised Ca^{2+} patients can get nephrocalcinosis and calculi. Hypertension also occurs. The hypercalcaemia causes constipation, peptic ulceration, pancreatitis and general malaise.

3.35 Parathyroidectomy **Answers: ABCE**

The best investigation is for an experienced parathyroid surgeon to explore both sides of the neck. Some surgeons would advocate the use of ultrasound, CT and radionucleotide scanning. Selective venous sampling has been used but not venography.

3.36 Congenital hypertrophic pyloric stenosis **Answers: DE**

This affects 4/1000 births, boys more frequently than girls. A positive family history is seen in 1 in 7 cases mostly on the maternal side. Persistent vomiting leads to hypochloraemic hypokalaemic alkalosis, requiring fluid replacement of 0.9% of saline with potassium. The diagnosis can be made by ultrasound or barium meal.

3.37 Parathyroidectomy **Answer: E**

The corrected calcium level and the symptoms of the patient should gauge the treatment of low calcium after parathyroid surgery. Simple supplementation is indicated in mild cases with oral calcium (Calcichew) with or without 1α cholecalciferol, the newer vitamin D supplement. For symptomatic disease (i.e. tingling around mouth and hand cramps) intravenous calcium should be used. (10 ml of 10% calcium gluconate given slowly diluted over 5 minutes.) The calcium levels should then be rechecked.

3.38 Pharyngeal web **Answers: BCDE**

Webs are more common in women and may be part of the Plummer-Vinson or Patterson-Kelly syndromes where the patient also has iron deficiency anaemia giving a microcytic picture. Webs and any upper constriction increase the incidence of aspiration.

3.39 Pharyngeal pouches **Answers: CDE**

Pharyngeal pouches may present with a mass in the anterior triangle of the neck which compresses and 'squelches'. The patient may be able to regurgitate at will. Recurrent overspill may cause pneumonia and if this occurs at surgery then the aspiration may lead to Mendelsohn's syndrome. In this condition there is a defect between the cricopharyngeus muscle and the thyropharyngeus (Killian's dehiscence). Surgery consists of excision of the pouch or suspension of the pouch now treated endoscopically via an incision anterior to the sternocleidomastoid muscle and a 3 cm cricopharyngeal myotomy.

3.40 Tonsillectomy **Answers: BC**

The indications for tonsillectomy are recurrent acute follicular tonsillitis (> 4 per year) or evidence of recurrent respiratory obstruction.

3.41 Mesenteric adenitis **Answers: BCE**

Mesenteric adenitis is caused by an adenovirus. There is often history of preceding upper respiratory tract infection with associated cervical lymphadenitis. There is typically a high fever (38°C) and poorly localised pain with no peritoneal signs. Treatment is conservative with simple analgesics.

3.42 Laryngeal carcinoma **Answers: DE**

Men (aged 60–70 years) are affected more significantly than women in the ratio of 6:1. Most laryngeal carcinomas develop on the vocal cords. Progressive voice change is the earliest sign. Stridor and dyspnoea are late features. Examination is performed by indirect laryngoscopy. Micro laryngoscopy is helpful when views are difficult or when a biopsy is needed. Radiotherapy alone may suppress local symptoms. In advanced disease radical radiotherapy is required. Curative treatment usually involves radiotherapy, surgery or a combination of the two.

3.43 Tonsillectomy **Answer: D**

Postoperative bleeding from the tonsillar bed occurs not infrequently and may respond to adrenaline soaked packs, however it frequently needs re-exploration. Although swallowing is painful post-operatively this does not lead to complete dysphagia. Secondary haemorrhage due to infection occurs in 1% of patients on days 5 to 8 and responds to antibiotics.

3.44 Lumps in the parotid gland **Answers: BDE**

Of the lumps presenting in the parotid region 90% will be salivary gland tumours and of these 90% will be adenomas, mostly pleomorphic. Pleomorphic adenomas are benign and behave benignly, however recurrences do occur post surgery due to incomplete excision on the finger-like projections of tumour. Facial nerve signs although not diagnostic are suggestive of malignant disease. All parotid tumours may have an increased incidence with radiation exposure.

3.45 Neonatal surgery **Answer: B**

The main problems associated with neonatal surgery are temperature control, nutrition and respiration. New-borns are very prone to hypothermia which together with opiate analgesia acts as a very strong respiratory depressant. All possible measures should be taken to reduce heat loss and the operating theatre should be kept above 25°C (30°C is too hot to work in!). The neonate can seldom absorb oral or nasogastric feed and so parenteral feeding is essential.

3.46 Oesophageal atresia **Answers: ABD**

Oesophageal atresia affects 1/3000 pregnancies and may be associated with tracheal atresia and tracheo-oesophageal fistulae. This condition forms part of the VACTERL syndrome (anomalies in Vertebrae, Anorectal, Cardiovascular, Tracheo-Esophageal, Renal, Limb). Ultrasound need not show an empty stomach if a fistula exists.

3.47 Tumours of the thyroid gland **Answers: AC**

Papillary thyroid carcinomas are four times more common in women than men. For a diagnosis of follicular carcinoma to be made vascular invasion or invasion into the capsule of the thyroid must be demonstrated, this is not possible using FNAC. Fine needle aspiration cytology however in experienced hands can diagnose medullary, anaplastic and papillary carcinomas. The results from the treatment of anaplastic thyroid carcinoma are almost universally poor. Radiotherapy may be used as palliation or with surgery. Isolated thyroid lymphoma should be treated with total thyroidectomy followed by radiotherapy.

3.48 Neonatal surgical conditions **Answers: BCDE**

3.49 Intussusception **Answers: BDE**

Intussusception usually presents between the age of 1 month to 1 year. The most common site is between the ileum and the colon although any site may intussuscept. Very rarely (< 10%) is a definite cause found although lymphoid hyperplasia in Payer's patches may play a role during a viral illness. The classical history is of bouts of screaming with the infant's legs being drawn up. Between these episodes the child is healthy. The child may pass 'redcurrant jelly' stool and may have a sausage shaped abdominal mass on examination. Diagnosis is made by ultrasound or barium studies which may be therapeutic.

4.1 Ileoanal pouch **Answer: E**

Selection of patients for a pouch is important as complications occur in 20–50% cases. Contraindications at present include those with Crohn's disease, particularly if there is any pelvic sepsis. Most surgeons routinely defunction to mitigate the effects of any pelvic sepsis. Pelvic sepsis occurs in approximately 30% of cases and is the most common complication of this procedure.

4.2 Abdominal obstruction **Answers: BCD**

The cardinal features are colicky central abdominal pain, abdominal distension and vomiting. The pain becomes constant if there is strangulation, ischaemia or perforation. Coffee-ground vomiting can occur but is unusual.

4.3 Bowel obstruction **Answers: BC**

The patients should have no oral intake. A nasogastric tube is important to empty the stomach. Resuscitation with intravenous fluids and analgesia are essential prior to surgery and night-time surgery is not commonly required. Albumin adds little.

4.4 Bowel obstruction **Answers: CE**

In large bowel obstruction the small bowel will still contain gas especially if the colon has decompressed via an incompetent ileo-caecal valve. The caecum distends the most in obstruction and due to Laplace's law will have the greatest tension in the wall causing ischaemia and perforation which occur most commonly when the caecal diameter is 10 cm. Vomiting is an early feature of small bowel obstruction.

4.5 Calot's triangle **Answers: BEF**

Calot's triangle is bounded by the free edge of the liver, the cystic duct and the common hepatic duct and contains the cystic node and the cystic artery.

4.6 Lesser omentum **Answers: AC**

The lesser omentum forms a free edge and the foramen of Winslow or aditus to the lesser sac, the portal vein lies most posterior with the artery to the left of the common bile duct. A double layer of peritoneum covers it. Squeezing this fold (Pringle's manoeuvre) reduces bleeding from the liver.

4.7 Small bowel obstruction **Answers: ABD**

The most likely cause will be adhesions from previous surgery but herniae, inguinal and femoral, are common. The history is incorrect for acute appendicitis and atresia will have presented earlier in infancy. Incisional hernias can obstruct although they usually have a wide neck. Intussusception is unlikely but possible and would usually be due to an intestinal tumour.

4.8 *Helicobacter pylori* eradication **Answers: ABE**

Sucralfate is used for dyspepsia but does not help in *H. pylori* eradication. Other drugs used include the other PPIs and H_2 antagonists together with tetracycline, erythromycin, clarithromycin and originally bismuth sulphate. Pirenzepine is a anticholinergic agent. Classically, triple therapy is used with two antibiotics with a proton pump inhibitor.

4.9 Upper GI bleed **Answers: ADF**

The initial management is resuscitation. In a patient such as the one described a central line should be used to guide aggressive fluid replacement monitored also by measuring urine output.

4.10 Surgery in upper gastrointestinal bleeds **Answers: ABDE**

Active bleeding on endoscopy can be injected with adrenaline or sclerosant; if this then fails and the patient rebleeds or fulfils the other criteria then surgery is essential. Uncontrollable bleeding at endoscopy will necessitate surgery.

4.11 Raised serum amylase **Answers: ADEF**

Small intestinal obstruction, diabetic ketoacidosis, mumps and abdominal trauma may also cause a raised serum amylase. Post ERCP pancreatitis and hence hyperamylassaemia is a well recognised complication.

4.12 Patients with acute pancreatitis **Answers: AE**

The mainstay of treatment is that of fluid resuscitation whether shocked or not. Pancreatitis is like a retroperitoneal burn and the patient therefore requires fluid replacement. For accurate replacement a urinary catheter should be inserted and in severe cases a central line. The patient will need a nasogastric tube and the analgesic of choice is pethidine. There is some debate about the use of antibiotics however the consensus at present is that they should be given in severe cases only (UK national guidelines 1998).

4.13 Removal of gallstones **Answers: ABDFG**

The most common way of solving this surgical problem today is the use of sphincterotomy and dredging at endoscopic retrograde cholangio-pancreatography, sometimes combined with lithotripsy. After an open exploration with or without choledochoscopy, a T tube is left in situ in the duct. After a delay this track can be dilated and stones flushed through or even retrieved percutaneously. The Burhenne technique involves the use of a steerable catheter passed down the mature T-tube track to retrieve retained stones. This is rarely used today as ERCP and duct clearance is achieved prior to cholecystectomy. Dissolution agents can have serious side-effects and so are no longer used.

4.14 Acute appendicitis **Answers: DEGH**

Symptoms or even a positive MSU do not exclude a diagnosis of acute appendicitis as the inflamed appendix can irritate the bladder. The WBC and even the temperature may be normal even in florid appendicitis. If the appendix is near the psoas muscle then it is painful to fully extend the right hip and forced extension is not possible. The Alvarado scoring system is used in the diagnosis of appendicitis.

4.15 Pyrexia **Answers: ABC**

The most common causes for a pyrexia this soon after surgery are basal atelectasis (especially common in smokers) and urinary tract infection possibly related to catheter insertion if the admission has been complex. If the patient has been in hospital for a few days with intravenous access then localised cellulitis around the cannula can cause pyrexia. At two days this is generally too early for a wound infection. An ileus per se will not cause a pyrexia.

4.16 Acute pancreatitis **Answers: BCD**

The amylase rise does not reflect severity; the WCC does however. (See Ranson Imrie criteria for assessing the severity of pancreatitis.) Patients often need insulin however in acute pancreatitis. Pancreatic supplements may be needed in chronic disease due to pancreatic insufficiency.

4.17 Anal fissure **Answers: CF**

Fissures cause classic pain on defaecation and after for a period of about 20 minutes. Chemical sphincterotomy may be achieved by the use of topical nitrates. If surgical sphincterotomy is performed it should be partial to maintain continence. Fissures occur in a posterior position in 80% of cases in men and 60% in women. Anal fissure is not a premalignant condition as opposed to anal condylomata which are related to anal carcinoma.

4.18 Angiodysplasia **Answers: BCE**

The most common site for this disorder is the right side of the colon. It may bleed massively and if the bleed is brisk enough then angiography may be helpful showing the site. A classic early draining vein may be evident on the angiogram.

4.19 Perianal abscess **Answers: BDE**

Perianal abscesses often start with an infection of the perianal glands causing an inter-sphincteric abscess. This then expands and may discharge and form a fistula. Fistulae, not abscesses, obey Goodsall's Law. Complex horseshoe abscesses may need MRI to assess them fully.

4.20 Pancreatic trauma **Answers: ABDE**

Pancreatic trauma is uncommon. It is most commonly due to blunt trauma with compression of the pancreas against the vertebral column. It most commonly occurs across the pancreatic neck and hence the duodenum and bile ducts may be injured. The essential component of making a diagnosis of pancreatic trauma is to consider the possibility as early as possible. A high concentration of amylase in diagnostic peritoneal lavage fluid may also be seen in small bowel perforation. CT should be performed followed by ERCP in equivocal cases.

4.21 Carcinoma of the gall bladder **Answers: ACD**

Carcinoma of the gall bladder has a 90% association with gallstones but overall it is a rare occurrence. The finding of carcinoma of the gall bladder is often seen at cholecystectomy. There is a very poor response to chemotherapy with the five year survival approaching 20% only.

4.22 Umbilical hernia **Answers: ABD**

At birth 10% of white children and 40% of Afro-Caribbean children have an umbilical hernia. The fascial defect is more common in premature infants. Conservative treatment is the rule especially if < 1 cm. Extraperitoneal fat is usually seen initially, omentum is also seen quite often. Chronic obstructive pulmonary disease is associated with direct inguinal hernia while ascites is associated with umbilical hernia.

4.23 Obturator hernia **Answers: BCD**

Obturator hernia occurs through the obturator canal. It is likely to strangulate because of the firm fibrous and bony edges around the neck. Commoner in women > 50 years. Presents with small bowel obstruction. Patients usually hold the affected hip joint in semi-flexion. The obturator sign (knee and hip are flexed to a right angle and the hip joint internally rotated) puts a stretch on the obturator nerve. A prolene mesh is used for the repair.

4.24 Colectomy for ulcerative colitis **Answers: ABCD**

A Kock pouch developed in 1969 is an internal ileal reservoir drained through the abdominal wall. Ileorectal anastomosis has the disadvantage that disease in the rectum remains to produce symptoms and may predispose to cancer. However, it does provide better continence than a pouch.

4.25 Proctitis **Answers: ABCE**

Inflammatory disease in the rectum may be caused by a number of microbial agents including *Mycobacterium tuberculosis* and *Treponema pallidum. Ascaris lumbricoides* usually gives rise to intestinal obstruction or appendicitis.

4.26 Haemorrhoids **Answers: CD**

Haemorrhoids are hypertrophied endoanal vascular cushions and not veins. Rectal varices occur in cirrhosis, which are distinct from haemorrhoids. Diet is very important in the treatment of haemorrhoids although banding and sclerosant injection of oily phenol (5% in almond oil and not 80% which is used in nail bed ablation for ingrowing toenails) have a role to play.

4.27 Carcinoma of the oesophagus **Answers: E**
The natural history of this malignancy is a progressive dysphagia for solids and then liquids with a loss of weight. It is most common in the lower third of the oesophagus. Recently adenocarcinoma has become more common than squamous cell carcinoma in the West. A chest film must be obtained to look for fistulation.

4.28 Right upper quadrant pain **Answers: ABDE**
Sickle cell disease is associated with pigment gallstones. Pelvic inflammatory disease can cause right upper quadrant pain especially due to *Chlamydia* (Curtis Fitz-Hugh), although this is rare.

4.29 Epigastric pain **Answers: ACDEF**
A variety of medical conditions can cause epigastric pain including diabetic ketoacidosis and ischaemic heart disease.

4.30 Diarrhoea **Answers: ABCDEF**
Chronic pancreatitis may cause diarrhoea which usually responds to exocrine pancreatic supplements. Patients post vagotomy may have diarrhoea due to motility changes. Codeine phosphate may cause overflow diarrhoea due to constipation.

4.31 Rectal cancer **Answers: CD**
The most important margin in any rectal excision is the lateral or circumferential margin and this forms the basis of total mesorectal excision. These cancers present with bleeding PR rather than right-sided tumours which classically present with anaemia. There is a degree of overlap between inflammatory bowel and cancer although patients with the former are usually younger. Preoperative radiotherapy may be used in those with operable tumours (one week of radiotherapy followed by surgery one week later) or in those with possibly inoperable tumours (four weeks of radiotherapy).

4.32 Ulcerative colitis **Answers: CE**
Ulcerative colitis is associated with backwash ileitis and has a 10% chance of malignant change at ten years increasing after that. Transmural inflammation occurs in Crohn's disease as does the cobble stone appearance (ulcerative colitis has ulcer formation and pseudo polyp formation).

4.33 Operating on a jaundiced patient **Answers: BCD**
The patient should be well hydrated and a forced diuresis may be created using the osmotic diuretic Mannitol to avoid hepatorenal syndrome and so renal failure. The patient's clotting should be normalised using vitamin K and fresh frozen plasma as needed.

4.34 Liver function **Answers: ABD**
The following may also be used: the transaminases, gamma GT and alkaline phosphatase enzyme levels.

4.35 Gallstones in the common bile duct **Answers: AD**
Cholecystostomy does not relieve common bile duct obstruction. Hepatico-docho-jejunostomy is not justified for benign disease but may be appropriate for malignant obstruction due to carcinoma of the pancreas.

4.36 Tender right iliac fossa **Answers: AB**
A perforated ulcer may present only with right iliac fossa pain especially if the presentation is delayed, the right iliac fossa is where the fluid accumulates. Ovulation may cause pain in this location in a woman. Acute pancreatitis will cause epigastric or generalised abdominal pain.

4.37 Right iliac fossa pain **Answers: ABCDE**
Tuberculosis may involve the caecum or cause a psoas abscess.

4.38 Peptic ulcer disease **Answers: ABCD**
Metformin has no associated risk, the others have. Also included in this list are the non-steroidal anti-inflammatory drugs. Blood group O is associated with peptic ulcer, whilst blood group A is associated with gastric carcinoma.

4.39 Posterior relations of the stomach **Answers: CDE**
Other relations include the left kidney and adrenal (not the right), the body and tail of the pancreas (not the head). The transverse mesocolon and the spleen are also relations.

4.40 Branches of the coeliac artery — Answers: CD

The coeliac axis gives rise directly to the hepatic, the left gastric and the splenic arteries. The hepatic then gives rise to the right gastric and the gastroduodenal arteries. The splenic artery gives rise to the short gastric arteries.

4.41 Obstructive jaundice — Answers: BCDEF

Gallstones in the gall bladder do not cause jaundice. A stone in the cystic duct may produce an inflammatory mass obstructing the common bile duct in the absence of a duct stone (the Mirizzi syndrome). Intravascular haemolysis causes prehepatic and not surgical jaundice (obstruction of the common bile duct). Colonic cancer may cause obstructive jaundice because of the primary tumour or because of metastasis to the liver or the hilar nodes.

4.42 Acholuric jaundice — Answers: BD

In acholuric jaundice there is a rise in unconjugated bilirubin and so the urine is a normal colour and the liver enzymes will be normal. Causes include haemolysis, blood disorders, massive haematomata and large tissue infarction. Steatorrhoea occurs in obstructive jaundice.

4.43 Hepatocellular jaundice — Answers: BDE

This type of jaundice causes dark urine, but not steatorrhoea, which is caused by obstructive jaundice. Transaminase enzymes are largely indicators of hepatic cellular function and so are raised. Alkaline phosphatase, however, predominantly rises in obstructive jaundice.

4.44 Indigestion — Answers: ABCE

Indigestion is a very broad symptom and means different things to different patients. One should always consider the rarer causes, for example, mesenteric ischaemia, especially if the pain is after meals and associated with a marked loss in weight.

4.45 Visceral pain — Answers: BD

Visceral pain is due to stretch receptors firing in response to strain on an organ or tube. It is poorly localised however it may be very distinctive enabling a diagnosis to be made.

4.46 Biliary colic **Answers: AB**

Biliary colic is not usually associated with pyrexia or a raised white blood count, these may indicate that the patient has cholecystitis. The duration of the pain is much longer (renal colic has this duration classically).

4.47 Blood supply of the oesophagus **Answers: E**

The inferior thyroid artery has branches that supply the oesophagus, but not the inferior phrenic artery. The thoracic aorta supplies the oesophagus throughout the chest.

4.48 Dysphagia **Answers: ABCDE**

Dysphagia may be due to a congenital web or Plummer-Vinson syndrome. A thoracic aortic aneurysm or a distended left atrium in mitral stenosis may also compress the oesophagus causing dysphagia.

4.49 Intra-thoracic oesophagus **Answers: ADE**

Relations include the right and left bronchi and the trachea, the vagus nerve, pleura, the arch and descending aorta and the thoracic duct.

4.50 Abdominal incisions **Answers: BD**

Midline incisions give quick good access and are associated with little blood loss, they have a poorer cosmetic result compared with transverse incisions. Paramedian incisions give good access however they are harder to make but can be more secure on closure (used routinely until the advent of synthetic non-absorbable sutures).

4.51 Ileostomy **Answers: BCE**

Chronic blood loss or vitamin B_{12} deficiency may give either anaemic picture. Bile salt loss due to an ileostomy may lead to the formation of gallstones.

4.52 Caecostomy **Answers: BE**

Caecostomy is occasionally used in an emergency to decompress an obstructed colon and may be used for colonic washout prior to an anastomosis. A loop ileostomy should be used to decompress the small bowel. The colon has no function in absorption of nutrients so caecostomy is of no value in feeding.

4.53 Truncal vagotomy — Answers: BDE

Truncal vagotomy fully removes all vagal stimulation to the stomach and so may cause stasis, alkaline gastritis, diarrhoea and early or late dumping syndromes.

4.54 Zollinger-Ellison (ZE) syndrome — Answers: All false

Gastrin levels are elevated in Zollinger-Ellison and rise on secretin administration. This syndrome may be treated with proton pump inhibitors.

4.55 Hepatomegaly — Answers: ABCE

Right ventricular failure can cause painful hepatomegaly as can congestive cardiac failure. Other causes include leukaemia and common bile duct obstruction.

4.56 Femoral herniae — Answers: AE

The hernia comes most medial with the vein on its lateral border. Femoral hernias are more prone to obstruction due to their small necks and are notoriously difficult to palpate.

4.57 Herniae — Answers: All false

Pain in a hernia may be for a variety of reasons including rapid expansion, infection or even malignant deposits within the sac. Small bowel is more likely to be found in a right sided hernia 2:1. The rectus sheath hernia is a Spigelian hernia.

4.58 A Kocher's incision — Answers: CEF

The fascia divided is Scarpa's fascia. T10 corresponds to the umbilical area. The rectus sheath is deficient posteriorly only below the arcuate line of Douglas but is present in two layers in the subcostal region.

4.59 Perforated duodenal ulcer — Answers: AE

In an emergency simple oversewing of the ulcer with an omental patch and washout of the abdomen is sufficient. There is no need for an ulcer biopsy in the duodenum (gastric ulcers should be biopsied however). Truncal vagotomy has fallen from favour in the emergency situation.

4.60 Acute cholecystitis **Answers: ACDE**

Either early cholecystectomy within three days of presentation or delayed after eight weeks or more is advocated. In the emergency situation an empyema can be drained via a cholecystostomy.

4.61 Charcot's triad **Answers: ACE**

Charcot's triad refers to the presentation of cholangitis and consists of fever, rigors and jaundice.

4.62 Lienorenal ligament **Answers: ACE**

Hypocalcaemia occurs as a result of chronic vomiting from pyloric obstruction. This leads to alkalotic hypochloraemia. Alkalosis may lead to reduced plasma raised Ca^{2+}. Resuscitation is carried out with normal saline with added K^{+}.

4.63 Gastric acid secretion **Answers: BD**

Gastrin, histamine, and acetylcholine increase gastric acid secretion; secretin, somatostatin and prostaglandins reduce it. The secretion occurs in three phases, namely cephalic, gastric and intestinal.

4.64 Complications of a chronic duodenal ulcer **Answers: ABDE**

4.65 Pancreatic pseudocysts **Answers: ABD**

Pseudocysts usually resolve spontaneously but if they do not resolve they can be treated percutaneously. After six weeks the cyst wall has thickened and this facilitates open cystgastrostomy. They may be drained through the stomach endoscopically. Internal drainage is preferable via a Roux loop to prevent pancreatic fistulae from forming. A pancreatic psuedocyst is a collection of fluid in the lesser sac.

4.66 Upper abdominal pain **Answers: ABCEF**

4.67 Epigastric pain **Answers: ACD**

A diagnosis needs to be made and the correct treatment instigated to resuscitate this man quickly and effectively. LFTs will only delay things and add little to the management. An ECG is essential to exclude cardiac ischaemia and pericarditis. Ultrasound is increasingly being performed in the A + E in the USA, but at present is not routine in the UK.

4.68 Oesophageal varices **Answers: ABCDE**
Varices if from cirrhosis have a 40% mortality which is much less if from an extrahepatic problem. They are porto-systemic anastomoses and may be treated either by intra- or para-vasal sclerosant injection.

4.69 Child's classification of portal hypertension **Answers: ABD**
Child's classification is into three grades using albumin, bilirubin, prothrombin time, the presence of ascites and encephalopathy.

4.70 Gastric erosions **Answers: ABDE**
A barium meal is not helpful in the diagnosis, which should be made on endoscopy although a barium meal may reveal ulcer disease.

4.71 Barrett's oesophagus **Answers: ACD**
Barrett's oesophagus refers to gastric metaplasia in the lower oesophagus. It is relatively common at endoscopy (up to 10%) and is pre-malignant. Proton pump inhibitors are usually effective in controlling inflammation although it may lead to both benign and malignant strictures.

4.72 Achalasia **Answer: BD**
Achalasia gives a bird's beak appearance on contrast studies, however dynamic films are needed and even then it can be difficult to make a diagnosis, endoscopy is still needed to exclude malignancy. The affected area has no peristalsis and may need a Heller's oesophagomyotomy, not Keller's operation for hallux valgus.

4.73 Perforation of the oesophagus **Answers: AB**
Boerhaave described perforation of the oesophagus after a large vomit. The treatment of perforated oesophagus depends upon the delay in presentation and the degree of contamination. Opinion varies. The patient should be kept nil by mouth and given parenteral nutrition, antibiotics and drainage of the chest cavity.

4.74 Gastro-oesophageal reflux disease (GORD) **Answers: ABDE**
Many of the symptoms of GORD respond to proton pump inhibitors (90%); failures to respond may be due to bile reflux.

4.75 Proton pump inhibitors (PPIs) Answer: B

Long term use of such drugs may lead to atrophic gastritis and apudomas. The first line of treatment is conservative with lifestyle changes such as cessation of smoking. PPIs may cause diarrhoea but this is rarely severe.

4.76 Oesophagitis Answers: DE

4.77 Herniae Answers: AC

The most common female adult hernia is a femoral, however taking all ages then inguinal herniae are more common. Inguinal herniae are more common on the right 5:4. Infant inguinal herniae are much more common in boys than in girls 8:1.

4.78 Herniae Answers: CE

Herniae are usually diagnosed clinically; only rarely in fat patients are other investigations needed for diagnosis. Richter's herniae strangulate but do not obstruct. Intra-abdominal malignancy may present with herniae either as direct transcoelomic spread or as a result of increased abdominal pressure from ascites. Direct and indirect herniae are difficult to distinguish clinically but this can easily be achieved at surgery by the lateral relationship of indirect herniae to the easily palpable inferior epigastric artery.

4.79 Inguinal canal Answers: BC

The deep ring is at the mid point of the inguinal ligament, the mid inguinal point is the surface marking for the femoral artery. In women the canal carries the round ligament of the uterus. In children it is very short as the internal and external rings lie almost on top of each other, with increasing age it elongates.

4.80 Ulcerative colitis Answers: ABE

Goblet cell/mucin depletion together with crypt abscesses are characteristic features of ulcerative colitis. Between the ulcers the surviving mucosa becomes swollen and hyperplastic forming polypoid excrescences.

4.81 Epigastric hernia **Answer: B**

An epigastric hernia is a protrusion of abdominal contents through the interstices between decussating fibres of the aponeuroses of the abdominal wall between the xiphoid process and the umbilicus. It is most common between the ages of 20 and 50. 20% are multiple but usually one is dominant. It usually contains preperitoneal fat and is closed directly unless very large when a mesh may be required.

4.82 Acute mesenteric ischaemia **Answers: ABCF**

Cardiac arrhythmias (especially atrial fibrillation), recent MI, hypotension due to pancreatitis or haemorrhage – all predispose to acute mesenteric ischaemia. There is a marked shift of intravascular volume into the bowel wall causing haemoconcentration and hypovolaemic shock. A high index of suspicion is required to identify acute mesenteric ischaemia. Sudden severe abdominal pain accompanied by rapid forceful bowel evacuation with minimal or no abdominal signs strongly suggests acute arterial occlusion.

4.83 Paraoesophageal hiatus hernia **Answers: ACDEF**

The symptom of dysphagia and post-prandial fullness is seen in paraoesophageal hernia as there is compression of the adjacent oesophagus by distended cardia or twisting of the gastro-oesophageal junction by torsion of the stomach. Respiratory complications are frequent. It is life threatening in 20% of cases and should be repaired electively.

4.84 Meckel's diverticulum **Answers: BDF**

A Meckel's diverticulum is a persistent remnant of the vitellointestinal duct. It occurs in 2% of the population, with a male:female ratio of 3:2. Usually 3–5 cm long and 10–50 cm from the ileocaecal valve. It possesses a mesentery but has an independent blood supply from the arcade of ileal vessels. There is no evidence that Meckel's diverticulum is an inherited trait but it is associated with other congenital malformations (especially exomphalos, oesophageal atresia). The lining of the diverticulum is the same as that of the ileum in most cases but may contain gastric, duodenal, colonic or pancreatic tissue (16% cases). About 4% lead to complications including haemorrhage (31%), inflammation (25%), bowel obstruction (16%), intussusception (11%) and hernia involvement (Littre's hernia).

4.85 Diverticulosis of the small bowel **Answers: BDE**

Solitary or multiple diverticula are usually found in the jejunum and less commonly in the ileum. Prevalence is in the order of 1%, on the mesenteric border but not invariably. Complications occur in < 10% cases: diverticulitis, perforation, haemorrhage, obstruction. Anaemia (due to vitamin B_{12} deficiency) can occur (blind loop syndrome).

4.86 Acute diverticulitis **Answers: ABD**

The incidence of diverticular disease increases with age. However, only 10% will become symptomatic. 90% of diverticula are located in the sigmoid colon and this is the exclusive site in 50%. When treated medically diverticulitis recurs in 25% with the majority of recurrences occurring in the first five years. CT scan with contrast is sensitive and specific with localised wall thickening > 5 mm, inflammation of pericolic fat and abscess formation. Gastrografin enema will show segmental lumen narrowing and tethered mucosa. Both investigations will show extraluminal air/gastrografin. A Hartmann's procedure is the safest option for perforation and faecal peritonitis. Colectomy and primary anastomosis has an 8% mortality, a 30% clinical leak rate and is not recommended for perforated diverticular disease or faecal peritonitis, however, some surgeons would perform such a procedure for purulent peritonitis.

4.87 Bile duct injury **Answers: BCE**

Bile duct injury following laparoscopic cholecystectomy has fallen to < 0.33%. If the cystic duct stump is not completely occluded by a clip, a biloma results. Complete clipping of the common bile duct leads to intrahepatic duct dilatation within days. Clinically significant strictures usually occur within weeks of the operation. Bile duct injury typically presents with RUQ pain caused by bile in the peritoneal cavity, with obstructive jaundice, peritonitis or septic shock. Ultrasound will show dilatation of the intrahepatic ducts. ERCP is the most useful test for the definitive diagnosis of major bile duct complications. Percutaneous transhepatic cholangiography can detect excluded duct segments caused by division or ligation of segmental ducts. CT may be important for detection of intraperitoneal bile and percutaneous drainage.

4.88 Carcinoid tumour of the appendix **Answer: AD**

Carcinoid tumour of the appendix is the most common of all tumours of the appendix. It is usually a solitary finding – occasionally associated with carcinoids of the ileum. 71% are found at the tip, 22% at the body and 7% at the base. The tumour may occur at any age but tends to affect patients in 30-40s. Metastatic spread is rare and thus carcinoid syndrome is uncommon. Carcinoid tumours < 2 cm are treated with appendicectomy and right hemicolectomy if > 2 cm.

4.89 Pseudomembranous colitis **Answers: BE**

Pseudomembranous colitis (PMC) is caused by *Clostridium difficile*. It is usually mild and self-limiting but occasionally may be severe and life-threatening. Many antibiotics may cause PMC but classically clindamycin and ampicillin. It is diagnosed either by biopsy, isolation of *Clostridium difficile* from faeces or direct demonstration of toxin. Sigmoidoscopy shows a characteristic membrane or grey/yellow material adhering to the colonic mucosa. The treatment involves stopping current antibiotic therapy and administering oral vancomycin or metronidazole.

4.90 Acute cholecystitis **Answers: ADEF**

Acalculous cholecystitis is unusual, occurring in 3% of cases. Aetiology of acute cholecystitis is unclear but is postulated to occur due to biliary stasis and increase in bile viscosity predisposing to irritation and inflammation of the gall bladder. Bacterial organisms are thought to play a secondary role in the pathogenesis of acute cholecystitis. Only in 20% of cases is a mass found, typically omentum overlying the gall bladder. Ultrasound has a sensitivity of over 95%. Diagnosis is suggested by shape, size, wall thickness and pericholecystic fluid collection. A sonographic positive Murphy's sign has an 85% correlation. Cystic duct obstruction represents the hallmark diagnosis of acute cholecystitis and is the basis of the HIDA scan.

4.91 Acute pancreatitis **Answers: ACD**

Acute pancreatitis is most commonly caused by gallstones (60% of cases). It is also recognised following stomach operations (1%). Ischaemic injury to the pancreas occurs in cardiopulmonary bypass. Hypoxia is seen in 40% patients in the first 48 hours – fall in inspiratory volume, decreased lung compliance, decreased diffusing capacity. Pseudocysts occur in 10% cases.

4.92 Acute pancreatitis **Answers: BDE**

Several scoring systems outlining early prognostic signs that correlate with the risk of major complications or death in acute pancreatitis have been described. The level of serum amylase does not correlate with the severity of the disease.

Age > 55,

WBC > 15 x 10^9/l	Glucose > 10 mmol/l
Albumin < 32 g/l	Urea > 16 mmol/l
PaO_2 < 8 kPa	LDH > 600 iu/l

AST > 200 iu/l.

The presence of three or more of the above criteria within the first 48 hours indicates a severe attack.

4.93 Colonic carcinoma **Answer: B**

Bile acids may act as carcinogens. Calcium in the diet binds bile acids, secondary bile acid secretion is raised after cholecystectomy. There is a 1 in 17 risk of death in individuals who have a single relative who has had colorectal cancer. Having a single first degree and single second degree relative affected gives a risk of 1 in 12. The incidence of synchronous colonic carcinoma is 3 to 5%. Up to 30% of patients have evidence of hepatic metastases at time of presentation and 5% pulmonary metastases.

4.94 Splenic flexure colonic carcinoma **Answers: ABCD**

Splenic flexure carcinoma has a high local recurrence rate and poor survival regardless of stage and presentation which may reflect surgical inadequacy of primary treatment.

4.95 Anal cancer **Answers: CE**

Anal cancer is uncommon, accounting for 4% of all large bowel malignancies. A history of genital warts (human papilloma viruses 6 and 11) increases the risk 25-fold. Human papilloma viruses 16, 18, 31 and 33 are commonly associated with genital condylomas but are more commonly found in high grade intra epithelial neoplasia and invasive carcinomas. Anal cancer spreads locally in a cephalad direction. Lymph nodes occur frequently but only 50% have tumour deposits. Pain and bleeding are the most common presenting symptoms.

4.96 Ulcerative colitis Answers: ADE

Ulcerative colitis most commonly presents with proctitis (bleeding and mucous secretion). Proximal extension of the disease (50% confined to rectum, 30% proctosigmoiditis and 20% beyond the splenic flexure). Granuloma formation is associated with Crohn's disease. In fulminant ulcerative colitis, all layers may be affected leading to perforation. Primary sclerosing cholangitis occurs in 4% cases.

4.97 Acute pseudocyts of the pancreas Answers: ABCE

Pancreatic pseudocysts are the most common cystic lesion of the pancreas and are collections of fluid in the lesser sac. They lack an epithelial lining. They occur in over 10% cases of pancreatitis as a result of duct disruption with leakage of pancreatic juice into the surrounding tissue. There is no natural border to the dissection of pancreatic juice, therefore pseudocysts may occur anywhere from the mediastinum to scrotum. Duct disruption may follow trauma. The most reliable means of making a diagnosis is via ultrasound or CT.

4.98 Chronic pancreatitis Answers: BCDE

Chronic pancreatitis is an inflammatory disease of the pancreas characterised by destruction of its exocrine and endocrine tissue and replacement with fibrous scar. The majority of cases are due to alcoholism. Gallstone pancreatitis is thought not to give rise to such widespread parenchymal destruction. Chronic pancreatitis usually occurs in men in their 30s. A rare autosomal dominant inheritance has been described whereby children 12–14 years of age develop chronic pancreatitis.

4.99 Chronic pancreatitis Answers: ACDE

Stopping alcohol ingestion improves pain in 50%. Pain relief should begin with small doses of oral medication such as codeine derivatives and working down the analgesic ladder. Operations to relieve pain are either 'drainage operations' to drain more adequately a dilated ductal system that is presumed obstructed or pancreatic resection to remove diseased tissue. Pancreaticojejunostomy will relieve pain in 80% of patients for the first several years.

4.100 Zollinger-Ellison syndrome **Answers: BCF**

Described in 1955 – severe peptic ulcer disease, hypersecretion of gastric acid and non-β islet cell tumour of pancreas. It occurs at all ages. 60% of gastrinomas are malignant. Most patients have ulcers in the duodenal bulb but multiple ulcers or in unusual locations should make one suspicious of Zollinger-Ellison syndrome especially if associated with diarrhoea. CT and angiography are the mainstay investigations. Control of gastric acid can be controlled by H_2 antagonists and proton pump inhibitors. Operative treatment includes curative resection of the gastrinoma and palliative reduction of tumour burden and gastrectomy.

4.101 Periampullary pancreatic carcinoma **Answers: ABDE**

Periampullary pancreatic carcinoma is usually a ductal adenocarcinoma. Rarely squamous, acinar and non-epithelial origin. Smoking is consistently associated with pancreatic carcinoma causing a two fold increased risk. FAP and Gardner's have duodenal polyps/adenocarcinoma as the most common extracolonic manifestation. CA 19–9 is usually elevated in pancreatic cancer and may be helpful in differentiating benign from malignant lesions.

4.102 Pancreatic pseudocysts **Answers: BCD**

Pancreatic pseudocysts are enzyme rich fluid collections in the lesser sac due to disruption of a pancreatic duct. The majority occur in alcoholic pancreatitis. Spontaneous rupture is associated with a 50% mortality. The cyst may be decompressed by drainage into the stomach or jejunum. Endoscopic cystduodenostomy has been used. Percutaneous drainage is performed for symptomatic cysts which do not communicate with the pancreatic system.

4.103 The spleen **Answers: AD**

The position of the spleen is in part maintained by several suspensory ligaments – gastrosplenic, splenocolic, splenophrenic and splenorenal. The gastrosplenic ligament contains the short gastric arteries. The capsule is normally 1–2 mm thick. The spleen is involved in haemopoiesis, storage and removal of Heinz bodies, Howell-Jolly bodies, removal of aged/abnormal RBCs. It is however an important reservoir for platelets.

ANSWERS – SYSTEM MODULE E: URINARY SYSTEM AND RENAL TRANSPLANTATION

5.1 Transurethral resection of prostate (TURP) Answers: CE

The indications for TURP rely on the man having outflow obstruction due to an enlarged prostate and repeated acute urinary retention with a failed trial without catheter. If his symptoms are debilitating or he has complications due to chronic retention then these are also an indication.

5.2 Prostatism Answers: ABCE

Prostatism presents with 1) obstructive symptoms, straining, poor stream, 2) irritation symptoms, urgency frequency and nocturia, 3) complications, renal failure, stones , infection. Tricyclic antidepressants and many neurological conditions such as spinal injury and Parkinsonism may cause sphincter disturbance and retention.

5.3 Blood in the urine Answers: BE

All blood in the urine is abnormal, anticoagulants may reveal pathology due to an increased bleeding tendency. Bleeding at the start of micturition may come from the urethra, blood at the end or throughout is usually due to a bladder or renal cause.

5.4 Renal function Answers: BDE

Urea levels will only rise after significant renal impairment and so are a poor indicator. Creatinine (produced by muscle) is only filtered and so clearance can give an estimate of renal clearance. Clearance may also be measured using EDTA (ethylene diamenetetra-acetic acid) labelled with ^{51}Cr or DTPA ^{99m}Tc (diethylenetriaminepenta-acetic acid labelled with technetium).

5.5 Renal adenocarcinoma Answers: BC

Renal adenocarcinoma usually presents after the age of 40 years, peaking at 65–75 years. 25–40% present with metastases (lung, liver, bone, brain). Only 10% have the classic triad of haematuria, loin pain and palpable loin mass. Renal carcinoma may give rise to paraneoplastic syndromes including weight loss, fever, erythrocytosis, hypercalcaemia (due to ectopic PTH production). Renal function is usually preserved. Tuberose sclerosis is associated with angiomyolipoma but not adenocarcinoma.

5.6 Wilms' tumour (nephroblastoma) Answers: ABD

It was first described in 1899 and found predominantly in children. 80% occur before age five years with the peak incidence at three years. 5% are bilateral. Sporadic cases occur in adults. 80% present with a palpable mass, 25% with haematuria and 30% with abdominal pain. 20% have metastases (lung and liver). The investigations include IVU, ultrasound and CT. Treatment involves surgery, radiotherapy and chemotherapy (actinomycin D). There is an 80% five-year survival.

5.7 Bladder cancer Answers: BE

Bladder cancer has a 3:1 male:female ratio and produces painless haematuria in the majority of cases (85%). Transitional cell carcinoma of the bladder arises predominantly from the posterior and posterolateral wall of the bladder. Bladder calculi can give rise to bladder cancer in the form of squamous carcinomas. Schistosomiasis is a major cause of bladder cancer especially in Egypt.

5.8 Urothelial TCC Answers: ABCDH

The incidence of urothelial carcinoma is 17 per 10^5 per annum. The male to female ratio is 3:1. The risk factors include smoking and occupational hazards (rubber, aniline dye and plastics). Haematuria is the most common symptom. The investigations of patients presenting with haematuria should include urine microscopy and culture, urine cytology, intravenous urography and cystoscopy. Intravesical mitomycin and BCG are used in the treatment of superficial TCC and carcinoma in situ of the bladder. Radical radiotherapy is indicated for invasive TCC in the elderly and for palliation.

5.9 Horseshoe kidney Answers: CDE

Horseshoe kidney is more common in men. The anatomical location and blood supply is very variable. They are more prone to infection and calculi formation due to relative upper tract stasis.

5.10 Renal cysts **Answers: ABE**

Cysts are present in 50% of patients over 70 years. They are usually painless and symptomless although they can cause pain or a mass. If found on an ultrasound scan, it can be seen if there is a solid component to the cyst (a sinister feature of malignancy). Aspiration should be performed for symptomatic cysts or ones in which there has been bleeding or rapid refilling, for diagnostic purposes. For cysts which continue to refill a de-roofing procedure may be carried out.

5.11 Ureteric injury **Answers: AB**

Ureteric injury is most commonly due to surgery and is often gynaecological. Other causes include external trauma, hyperextension injury of the spine. The best results are obtained when the injury is recognised early. Delayed recognition results in ureteric obstruction or development of a fistula. Primary direct repair can be performed using absorbable sutures if there is good blood supply and no tension. All repairs require internal splintage with a double J stent (for at least ten days) and external drainage. A Boari bladder flap is used to repair lower 1/3 ureteric injuries.

5.12 Genito-urinary tract trauma **Answers: ACDE**

10% of all patients with abdominal injuries have associated injuries of the urinary tract. The most important indicator is the presence of blood in the urine. Blood is present in 60% of patients with renal injuries and in all patients with bladder or urethral injuries. An absent nephrogram on IVU may suggest congenital agenesis but may be a sign of severe injury to the renal vasculature.

5.13 Prostatic adenocarcinoma **Answers: BCF**

The lifetime risk of developing prostatic cancer is 10%. Haematogenous spread occurs predominantly to bone (sclerotic lesions) and lymphatic spread occurs to pelvic lymph nodes. The clinical features include bladder outflow obstruction, bony pain due to metastases and haematuria.

5.14 Ovarian cancer **Answers: ACD**

Ovarian cancer accounts for 25% of all gynaecological malignancies. The risk factors include late menopause, nulliparity, late first pregnancy, peritoneal talc use and family history of ovarian, endometrial, breast or bowel cancer. Debulking surgery followed by chemotherapy (cisplastin and cyclophosphamide and more recently Taxol) is the mainstay of management. Radiotherapy has a role in the management of recurrent disease. The five-year survival rate varies from 88% for stage I to 20% for advanced disease.

5.15 Testicular neoplasms **Answers: AD**

The majority of testicular neoplasms occur in men under 40. Trucut and FNA are usually avoided for fear of scrotal tumour implantation and, for the same reason, surgery is carried out through an inguinal approach. Good survival figures of 80% and above are achieved but only by combination of surgery, radiotherapy and chemotherapy as the tumours frequently have pelvic lymphatic metastases at the time of presentation.

5.16 The bladder **Answers: BC**

The bladder has peritoneum covering its superior surface and is reflected anteriorly onto the abdominal wall. It is separated from the rectum by a thick fibrous layer (fascia of Denonvilliers), it is much thinner in the female. The ureters enter the bladder posteriorly at its base and run obliquely through the muscle and mucosal layers for 1.5–2 cm. The bladder receives its blood supply from the internal iliac artery – superior and inferior vesical arteries.

5.17 Prostate carcinoma **Answers: AB**

Prostate carcinoma usually affects men between 65–85 years. It is rare in Japan. Typically, prostatic carcinoma arises in the periphery of the posterior part of the prostate from an isolated nodule or diffuse involvement. It spreads initially by local extension, lymphatic spread to the pelvic nodes and haematogenous spread chiefly to the axial skeleton (particularly lumbar spine and pelvis) via Batson's valveless vein. Blood borne spread to other sites such as lung and liver is occasionally seen. The staging is T1: no tumour palpable, T2: tumour confined within the prostate, T3: extension beyond the capsule, T4: fixed to neighbouring structures.

5.18 Polycystic renal disease **Answers: ABCE**

There are two forms of this disease: the recessive infantile form and the dominant adult type. In the infantile form cystic changes occur in the kidneys and the liver. Portal hypertension may ensue leading to oesophageal varices. The adult form presents with renal failure in the third or fourth decade.

5.19 Ureteric duplication **Answers: CE**

Ureteric duplication is usually isolated to one side. The lower pole ureter enters the bladder superiorly and so it has a relatively short submucosal course compared with the upper pole ureter. It is for this reason that the lower pole ureter refluxes more often. The main problems seem with reduplication are reflux and recurrent infection.

5.20 Renal trauma **Answers: BC**

The findings of renal trauma are associated with an absent psoas shadow, and enlarged kidney, fractures of ribs 10, 11, 12 or the transverse processes of T2 or T3. Scoliosis may also be present to the injured side. Riggler's sign indicates free intra-abdominal gas.

5.21 Acute pyelonephritis **Answers: ABC**

Acute pyelonephritis is like any other acute infection. The patient is febrile with a tachycardia and features of infection. The patient may have a history of dysuria or frequency. Renal failure may be a late sequel to chronic infection and reflux.

5.22 Metastatic prostate carcinoma **Answers: ABCG**

Metastatic disease is treated by hormonal manipulation although some doubt remains about when this should be commenced. In symptomatic metastases immediate hormone manipulation should be started. Treatment may include orchidectomy, anti-androgens (cyproterone acetate, flutamide) and gonadotrophin releasing hormone analogues (buserelin, goserelin) which inhibit release of LH responsible for stimulating testicular production of testosterone.

5.23 Testicular seminoma **Answers: AE**

The clinical features of seminoma include testicular pain, scrotal mass, secondary hydrocele, lymphadenopathy, gynaecomastia and symptoms due to metastases. Orchidectomy through an inguinal approach usually confirms the diagnosis of testicular cancer. The suspicion of testicular cancer is a contraindication to FNAC and cone biopsy. Such investigations carry the risk of dissemination along the needle track and scrotal wall disease which is difficult to control. The tumour is sensitive to radiotherapy and chemotherapy (carboplatin and etoposide).

5.24 Testicular seminoma **Answers: ABCDE**

Testicular seminoma usually presents with a painless swelling in the scrotum. 10–15% patients present with a story of an injured testicle. Seminomas and teratomas secrete hCG causing gynaecomastia or mastitis. Seminomas are very radio-sensitive. Radiotherapy forms the basis of treatment together with orchidectomy.

5.25 Carcinoma of the penis **Answer: B**

Squamous cell carcinoma of the penis occurs in uncircumcised men. Circumcision affords some degree of protection against penile carcinoma if performed before puberty. Inguinal lymph nodes are involved in 50–60% cases but in half of these it is a result of secondary infection and not nodal metastases. Stage I and II lesions can be treated with radiotherapy alone. When the disease is extensive involving the iliac nodes the prognosis is dismal.

5.26 Priapism **Answers: ACDE**

Priapism is the condition whereby the penis remains erect despite the absence of sexual stimulation. The erection is confined to the corpora cavernosa. It is seen in patients with leukaemia, pelvic malignancy, perineal trauma and alcohol abuse. The treatment is initially aspiration of the corpora followed by injection of metaraminol (sympathetic amine causing vasoconstriction). If this fails then embolisation of the pudendal vessels and a corporasaphenous shunt are other options.

5.27

A	renal carbuncle	5.	ultrasound drainage
B	acute pyelonephritis	3.	antibiotics
C	chronic pyelonephritis	1.	hypertension
D	pyonephrosis	2.	nephrostomy
E	perinephric abscess	4.	incision and drainage

5.28 Renal TB **Answers: AD**

TB can affect any part of the renal tract from the kidney to the urethra. It is more common in men and usually presents in the patient's 40s or 50s. It usually presents with frequency. (Dysuria only if there is secondary infection.) Haematuria and pain occur if the upper tracts are obstructed due to caseation and disease spread. Treatment is with anti-tuberculous therapy. The patient should be closely followed and the obstructive symptoms should be sought and treated with stenting if they occur.

5.29 Ureteric obstruction **Answers: ABCE**

Inflammatory bowel disease may cause obstruction as can any process causing fibrosis of the surrounding area to the ureters. Aneurysmal disease of the aorta and retroperitoneal fibrosis can cause obstruction.

5.30 Renal tract calculi **Answers: ABE**

Stones are more common in people with a high protein diet. The presence of reflux and chronic infection together with impaired drainage all lead to an increased rate of stone formation. The majority of the calculi are composed of calcium oxalate (75%). The rest are mixed phosphate, urate and a minority are cysteine and xanthine.

5.31 Undescended testis **Answers: DE**

The full term incidence is about 2% but in premature infants it rises to approximately 20%. The most common site for maldescent is the superficial inguinal pouch. It is more common on the right than on the left. The risk of seminoma is in the region of 40x increased risk. Surgery must be performed before two years of age to preserve function. Testes found at the base of the penis are ectopic and not undescended.

5.32 Torsion of the testis **Answers: ADE**

Testicular torsion presents with acute scrotal, lower abdominal or hip pain. Predisposing factors include maldescended testis, transverse lying testis and long mesorchium. Ultrasound is only an adjunct to the diagnosis. The definitive and only reliable method of ensuring the correct diagnosis is surgical exploration. A torsion is repaired either by invaginating the tunica vaginalis and fixing the testis to the dartos muscle or by the Jaboulay technique. The opposite testis must also be fixed. If operated on within 5 hours 80% are viable. After 24 hours all twisted testes are infarcted.

5.33 Nephroblastoma **Answers: ACE**

Nephroblastoma or Wilms' tumour is embryologically associated with hypospadias and hemihypertrophy of the body. It represents 12% of the childhood cancers and presents at the age of one to three years. The presentation is of a painless abdominal mass associated with failure to thrive, haematuria and pyrexia. The treatment is radical surgery with chemo-radiotherapy.

5.34 Renal cell carcinoma **Answers: ACD**

Renal cell carcinoma (clear cell) is more common in men. There is an association with smoking, coffee ingestion, lead, asbestos and aromatic hydrocarbons. The spread of these very vascular tumours is via the blood stream and tongues of tumour can advance up the renal vein to the IVC and the heart.

5.35

A	acute rejection	2.	cellular immunity
B	hyperacute rejection	4.	pre-sensitisation
C	chronic rejection	1.	humoral system
D	blood group mismatch	3.	haemolysis

5.36 Idiopathic scrotal oedema **Answers: BCE**

Idiopathic scrotal oedema is an acute oedematous swelling of the scrotal skin usually occurring in boys younger than five years. The cause is unknown. Swelling may affect both sides of the scrotum and often into the thigh and groin. The scrotal contents are normal and there is a pink colour to the skin. It is a clinical diagnosis and management is conservative.

5.37 Acute epididymitis **Answers: ABDE**

Acute epididymitis is seen in all age groups but is rare before puberty. The infection reaches the epididymis via the bloodstream or retrograde from the prostatic urethra and seminal vesicles. Predisposing factors include UTI, STD infection and instrumentation of the urethra. *E. coli* is responsible for most infections. Late infection may be impossible to differentiate from torsion of the testis. In the long-term, atrophy of the testis occurs in 20% of patients and fertility may be impaired.

5.38 Acute renal failure **Answers: ADE**

In acute renal failure the kidney is not able to perform its normal functions. It does not concentrate urine and is unable to reabsorb sodium or excrete urea.

5.39 Urethral stricture **Answers: ABCDE**

There are many complications from a urethral fistula. Retention, infection, periurethral abscess, calculi due to stagnation and infection, diverticulae and fistulae. Malignant change may occur. The straining can lead to herniae and rectal prolapse. The constant back pressure may lead to renal failure, this then can lead to secondary hyperparathyroidism.

5.40 Hypospadias **Answer: B**

Hypospadias is the most common abnormality of penile development (1:400 live births) and is due to imperfect fusion of the genital folds and the glanular urethra. The optimum age for correction is 15–18 months (treatment completed before genital awareness and before the child needs to stand to void at school). The aim of treatment is to allow the patient to void with a forward pointing stream and to have a penis that is straight on erection and outwardly normal in appearance.

5.41 Bladder calculi **Answers: BCD**

Bladder calculi usually arise *de novo* in the bladder as a result of bladder outflow obstruction, diverticula or foreign bodies. The classical picture is of sudden cessation of urinary stream during voiding with severe penile/perineal pain. Bladder calculi may be treated with extracorporeal shock wave lithotripsy (ESWL) but more commonly by endoscopic removal.

5.42 Ectopic testes **Answers: BCD**

It is important to differentiate between ectopic and undescended. The deep inguinal ring and the superficial inguinal ring are positions where the testicle can be found but these are undescended and not ectopic.

5.43 Testicular torsion **Answers: CD**

The age of presentation is 14 to 20 years. If the testicle is high and hanging horizontally (clapper bell testes) then it is more likely to twist.

5.44 Prostate gland **Answers: BDE**

Benign prostatic hypertrophy occurs mainly in the periurethral zone. As this expands with whorls of nodular hyperplasia it compresses the gland to form a pseudo capsule. The other changes of atrophy, infection and malignancy, mainly occur in the postero-lateral peripheral zone.

5.45 Complications of TURP **Answers: BCD**

The complications of TURP include hypothermia and transurethral syndrome. In the latter, absorption of the hypotonic irrigation solution leads to water intoxication and causes intra-vascular haemolysis, hyponatraemia and hypotension. Other complications include: urethral stricture, incontinence (due to residual bladder instability), retrograde ejaculation and increased risk of myocardial infarct three years post TURP.

5.46 Prostatic cancer **Answers: ABC**

Prostatic cancer is rare before the age of 50. It may present as acute retention of urine or blood in the urine or sperm. It may present at an advanced stage with bony secondaries and pelvic lymph nodes.

5.47 Seminoma of the testis **Answers: ADE**

Seminoma of the testis accounts for 40% of testicular tumours with peak incidence between 30–40 years. The testis is symmetrically enlarged and the tumour is well demarcated with a creamy white appearance. Haematogenous spread occurs late in seminoma. Seminoma is extremely radiosensitive and remains the treatment of choice in early small volume disease. Chemotherapy is used for bulky or advanced metastatic disease (cisplatin). Overall survival is excellent.

5.48 Teratoma of the testis **Answers: ADE**

Teratoma of the testis has an earlier peak incidence than seminoma (20–30 years). There is a history of trauma in 20% cases. Haematogenous spread is early in teratoma of the testis. α-fetoprotein and β-hCG have both proved useful tumour markers in teratoma. 73% of patients with teratoma have elevated plasma levels of one or both markers.

5.49 Renal calculi **Answers: CD**

Renal calculi usually present in early adult life with two age peaks at 28 and 55 years. Common identifiable causes include idiopathic hypercalciuria (65%) and UTI (20%). Infective stones are staghorn calculi (Ca^{2+}, Mg^{2+}, NH_4PO_4) – formed by enterobacteria such as *Proteus* which produces urease that splits urinary urea to form ammonium ions. Renal pelvic stones, if symptomatic and large, require ESWL, percutaneous nephrolithotomy or nephrectomy.

5.50 Extracorporeal shock wave lithotripsy **Answers: CDE**

ESWL can be used for all stones except for cysteine stones which are very hard. Stones in the upper and lower 1/3 of the ureter may be treated with ESWL. The push–bang technique is used for stones in the upper 1/3 of the ureter.

5.51

A	aminoglutethamide	5.	use with prednisolone
B	cyproterone acetate	1.	anti-androgen
C	goserelin	4.	GnRH analogue
D	stilboestrol	2.	oestrogen
E	tamoxifen	3.	use in breast cancer

INDEX

Numbers given refer to the relevant question number. The word shown may not always be used in the question, but may appear in the explanatory answer.

Index

PASTEST COURSES

PASTEST: the key to exam success, the key to your future.
PasTest is dedicated to helping doctors to pass their professional examinations. We have 25 years of specialist experience in medical education and over 3000 doctors attend our revision courses each year.

Experienced lecturers:
Many of our lecturers are also examiners and teach in a lively and interesting way in order to:
✓ reflect current trends in exams
✓ give plenty of mock exam practice
✓ provide essential advice on exam technique

Outstanding accelerated learning:
Our up-to-date and relevant course material includes MCQs, colour slides, X-rays, ECGs, EEGs, clinical cases, data interpretations, mock exams, vivas and extensive course notes which provide:
✓ hundreds of high quality questions with detailed answers and explanations
✓ succinct notes, diagrams and charts

Personal attention:
Active participation is encouraged on these courses, so in order to give personal tuition and to answer individual questions our course numbers are limited. Book early to avoid disappointment.

Choice of courses:
PasTest has developed a wide range of high quality interactive courses in different cities around the UK to suit your individual needs.

What other candidates have said about our courses:
'Absolutely brilliant - I would not have passed without it! Thank you.'
Dr Charitha Rajapakse, London.
'Excellent, enjoyable, extremely hard work but worth every penny.'
Dr Helen Binns, Oxford.

For further details contact PasTest on

FREEPHONE 0800 980 9814

PasTest, FREEPOST, Knutsford, Cheshire WA16 7BR, UK.
Fax: 01565 650264 e-mail: courses@pastest.co.uk
web site: http://www.pastest.co.uk